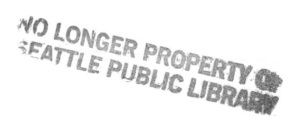

LIGHTNING FLOWERS

LIGHTNING FLOWERS

FLOWERS

MY JOURNEY TO UNCOVER THE COST

OF SAVING A LIFE

KATHERINE E. STANDEFER

Little, Brown Spark

New York Boston London

Copyright © 2020 by Katherine E. Standefer

Little, Brown Spark
Hachette Book Group
1290 Avenue of the Americas, New York, NY 10104
littlebrownspark.com

First Edition: November 2020

Little, Brown Spark is an imprint of Little, Brown and Company, a division of Hachette Book Group, Inc. The Little, Brown Spark name and logo are trademarks of Hachette Book Group, Inc.

The Hachette Speakers Bureau provides a wide range of authors for speaking events. To find out more, go to hachettespeakersbureau.com or call (866) 376-6591.

ISBN 978-0-316-45036-2
LCCN 2020936927

1 2020

LSC-C

Printed in the United States of America

To the girl in the parking lot:
Here is the book you needed.

CONTENTS

Prologue *Tucson, Arizona, 2012*   1

PART I: THE REVEALING

Chapter 1 *Boulder, Colorado, 2007*   5
Chapter 2 *Jackson, Wyoming, 2009*   15
Chapter 3 *Sylmar, California, 2013*   38
Chapter 4 *Boulder, Colorado, 2009*   49
Chapter 5 *Moramanga, Madagascar, 2014*   67
Chapter 6 *Maroseranana, Madagascar, 2014*   88
Chapter 7 *Boulder, Colorado, 2009*   97
Chapter 8 *Boulder, Colorado, 2010*   104
Chapter 9 *Boulder, Colorado, 2010*   111
Chapter 10 *Tucson, Arizona, 2012*   131
Chapter 11 *Fort Dauphin, Madagascar, 2014*   146

PART II: THE DISMANTLING

Chapter 12 *Tucson, Arizona, 2016*   163
Chapter 13 *Busoro, Rwanda, 2016*   196
Chapter 14 *Tucson, Arizona, 2017*   204
Chapter 15 *Rochester, Minnesota, 2017*   227

Epilogue   241
Acknowledgments   251
Index   259

In the name of which love should I act and how should I act? In the name of which love should I sacrifice another love? Whom shall I love the most and to whom do the most good—to my wife, or to my children; —to my wife and children, or to my friends? How shall I serve a beloved country without doing injury to the love for my wife, children, and friends? Finally, . . . to what extent can I occupy myself with my own affairs and yet be able to serve those I love?

—Leo Tolstoy,
On Life

I can only answer the question "What am I to do?" if I can answer the prior question "Of what story or stories do I find myself a part?"

—Alasdair MacIntyre,
After Virtue

The knowledge of death is reflective and conceptual, and animals are spared it. They live and they disappear with the same thoughtlessness: a few minutes of fear, a few seconds of anguish, and it is over. But to live a whole lifetime with the fate of death haunting one's dreams and even the most sun-filled days—that's something else.

—Ernest Becker,
The Denial of Death

LIGHTNING
FLOWERS

For centuries philosophy has taught that there are four causes:

(1) the *causa materialis*, the material, the matter out of which, for example, a silver chalice is made; (2) the *causa formalis*, the form, the shape into which the material enters; (3) the *causa finalis*, the end, for example, the sacrificial rite in relation to which the chalice required is determined as to its form and matter; (4) the *causa efficiens*, which brings about the effect that is the finished, actual chalice, in this instance, the silversmith....

The four causes are the ways, all belonging at once to each other, of being responsible for something else.... The three previously mentioned ways of being responsible owe thanks to the pondering of the silversmith for the "that" and the "how" of their coming into appearance and into play for the production of the sacrificial vessel.

    —Martin Heidegger, "The Question Concerning Technology"

PROLOGUE

N othing can prepare you for what it feels like to be shocked by an implanted cardioverter defibrillator. Like a badly spliced film reel, my memory of the night is fractured: in one instant, a player on the other intramural soccer team had fallen and the game stopped; he was getting up, brushing his thighs. In the next, my hands became claws. A maul cracked open my chest with a sickening thump, a hot whip tearing through my back. *Did somebody kick in my spine?* And then I knew. And I was screaming.

"There's no way you wouldn't scream if you felt it," my sister had said.

By then, the defibrillator had been in my body for three silent years, resting loyally above my left breast, keeping watch for the arrhythmia that could send me to the ground unconscious, with a heart quivering rather than pumping blood.

Now, on a crisp November night in Tucson, Arizona, I dropped to my knees in time for the second shock. *What if it doesn't stop?* I knew something was wrong, either with my device or with my body, but probably my ICD. If it was an arrhythmia, I should have been collapsed, unconscious—not sharp and alive like this, staring at the backs of houses at the edge of the field, their kitchen lights spilling dully out the windows as I screamed. "Call 911!"

A third shock. *You can either scream or breathe,* a voice inside me said, and I began to pull in air, cold heavy breaths, the way I'd learned to breathe into pain in yoga. *I am either alive or dead, and I choose which.*

The device did not fire again.

"Can I get someone behind me?" I called out. "I don't trust myself not to fall." Someone cupped my back immediately, supported me to the ground, and the sky came into view. A ring of faces. The sharp white field lights.

The smell of burning, which was me.

There is a kind of dream state that settles over the body in these moments, a clarity that rarely visits us when our lives are busy unfolding. For lying on my back, looking at the stars, a question lodged itself in my brain, a wild constellation of if-then statements.

If the defibrillator just saved my life. If a defibrillator is just metal. If metal is mined earth. If children sometimes work in mines, if tunnels collapse, if warlords profit, if women are raped, if mountains are dismantled and made toxic.

If mined earth just saved my life: Was it worth it?

The thin, branched burns that uncoil from the heads and necks of lightning-strike victims are sometimes called lightning flowers. Fernlike, following the patterns of rain or sweat, they are rose-colored lightning bolts frozen onto the body, as beautiful as they are terrible.

I will never know what my insides looked like after two thousand volts—if my tissue erupted into lightning flowers of the body cavity, a sudden bloom. What I do know is that the night I took three shocks to the heart I was marked, called into the world in a way I could not turn away from.

What can save us, I would learn, never comes without cost.

Some people say lightning strikes cure blindness; this is my version.

PART I
THE REVEALING

CAUSA FINALIS

CHAPTER 1

Boulder, Colorado
2007

The first time my younger sister passed out, she was eighteen, just beginning her freshman year of college at the University of Colorado in Boulder. One hungover morning in her dorm room in the fall of 2007, her phone rang, and she muted the call. She was sliding the phone back underneath her pillow when she blacked out and tumbled off the bed.

When she woke, everything was blurry, dreamlike. Her fan loud and big as a train. Christine's roommate found her crumpled on the dorm-room floor and raced for the resident assistant, who called 911. At the hospital, doctors checked her blood sugar, took a CT scan to look for epilepsy. Nothing was conclusive, so as the months ticked quietly on—football games and classes, mountain hikes and parties— her strange fall out of bed receded from view.

Then in December, just days before finals, it happened again. This time her roommate's phone went off, and she fell back into her pillow. When Christine came to, she called our parents in the Chicago suburbs, who began setting appointments for her over winter break. She would, after all, be home in just a few days.

Instead my sister, by then nineteen, spent those few days going into cardiac arrest over and over—first in the campus health center, then in the hospital, where a nurse noticed an abnormality in her heartbeat that pointed toward a dangerous genetic condition. The first time my parents received a call from a cardiologist named Dr. Sameer Oza at Boulder Community Hospital, he told them he could not release their daughter until she had a cardioverter defibrillator implanted. Christine had a rare arrhythmia, he told them, one that seemed to be activating cardiac arrest when she was startled. She had been lucky so far—her heart had restarted itself each time—but she might not be so lucky in the long term.

My parents bought plane tickets. Meanwhile my sister—surprised by a nurse in her doorway at the hospital—discovered the ceiling tiles spinning and woke suddenly with paddles poised above her chest.

"I have been dead," she told me years later.

Picture the sign posted on the door of her hospital room: DO NOT STARTLE THE PATIENT. SPEAK SOFTLY. And my mother creeping into the room whispering, "Christine, Christine."

I don't remember getting the call that she was in the hospital, but I do remember crying for her. That winter I lived in a one-room cabin on the property of a summer camp south of Jackson, Wyoming, five miles past the Hoback Junction, in a small valley rimmed by dark pine forests, where cliffs hung off the mountains like broken teeth. On the Broken Arrow Ranch, we had woodstoves, no cell service, and a bridge across the pale blue tongue of the Hoback River, which was slowly hardening into swaths of ice. The week my sister almost died in the Colorado foothills, we were deep in mud season up in Wyoming, tree roots jutting up at angles out of the first paltry snowbanks, trails slippery with melt. We'd already had a freeze over Thanksgiving that left my toilet tank solid.

It was the beginning of a life I'd dreamed of since childhood. I'd grown up in a suburb northwest of Chicago—not one of the leafy old towns along the lake, with their grand brick estates and quaint downtowns, but a subdivision farther out, forty-five minutes down the train line, where the trees were just gaining height, on land that had until the early 1960s been a tomato farm. All down my block, a few standard split-level and colonial houses repeated, each with different-colored shutters and brick facades, their grass trimmed, flowers blooming in rows every spring.

These were the years of expansion; these were the decades of sprawl. What had once been tallgrass prairie edged by forest, with bluestem so dense the horizon wavered, now disappeared beneath strip malls and subdivisions, until my neighborhood was sentineled by big-box stores and their vast parking lots. The concrete stretched most of the way to the Wisconsin border. And though I loved the way tornado winds blew off the plains into Chicagoland each May—ominous green-gray thunderheads crackling over the softball fields—these twists of wildness were rare. Most often the uniformity settled over me like a stranglehold. The flat gray of the sky during Chicago's seemingly endless winter; the stifling humidity of summers that left the house sticky. All around me I saw a place being plucked and prodded into form, the wild-growing plants weeded out. The deer that had once ghosted the scrap of wetland at the end of our street disappeared when more McMansions went in. Even as a child, despair filled me whenever I saw a SOLD sign on a wooded lot by the side of the road. I knew what came next, and I felt the loss in my very body.

When my parents first brought the three of us girls out West, I was in preschool, and though I spent as much time throwing up from altitude sickness as I did strapped into my tiny plastic ski boots, something of the big white massifs, the unruly pale rivers, imprinted in me. At first we went to Colorado every other year; by late elementary school, the trips were yearly, and each time the minivan turned east again I found myself weeping, leaned over the back seat to watch the mountains recede. All that crisp sun, all those big views, the miles with nothing in sight but a ranch house or two. Afternoons spent in the company of deep snow and pine trees. I had found something there. The first year we drove through the Nebraska panhandle on our way to northern Colorado, crossing the barren stretch of highway from Cheyenne, Wyoming, into the Medicine Bow, I was seven. Those sagebrush steppes, the pulse and push of the wind, the dirt roads that twisted away. I began to say it aloud with the kind of knowing that seven-year-olds can have: I would become a writer in a cabin in Wyoming.

The fall Christine began passing out, I had just graduated from college down in Colorado Springs. By then I'd spent many summers in Jackson

Hole and the less-tracked mountains to the south and east—arriving in late spring blizzards, leaving as the aspens turned yellow. I'd been a student, then staff, at a wilderness school. I spent my winters heavy with longing for the place: its silver storms, its antelope, its bear. That first summer out of college, I worked for the camp that owned the Broken Arrow Ranch, and when the place emptied out, I moved into tiny Cabin 2. For the first time, I had an address in Wyoming good for more than a summer. The month Christine first went into cardiac arrest in her dorm room, I was roving the dense woods behind the ranch, stockpiling kindling for the winter. I'd bought a little axe and a sizable maul and a couple of wedges, and under a pine beside my house I was learning to split wood. By the time Dr. Oza leveled his ultimatum at my parents in December, I was training to be a ski instructor—driving seventeen miles north to town each morning before hopping on a bus to the resort, where on the slopes of the Tetons we practiced holding a wedge position on a single strip of icy man-made snow. It was not a job I'd dreamed of consciously, but when a woman leaned over the desk at the climbing gym where I worked to tell me she was applying, it made sense. I was broke, living on ramen and tuna sandwiches, still trying to figure out how things would work for me. And if the land itself had called me all these years, outdoor adventure sports became the paycheck that allowed me to stay. Being a ski instructor would round out the year, allowing me more space to write during mud season—those weeks between summer and snow, snow and summer, when town shut down. Now my winter work would rise with the flow of tourists into town—peaking with required three-week-long, no-days-off stretches around Christmas and spring break—and ebb just when I couldn't take it anymore, leaving me, ideally, with a reasonable bank account and weeks of open space to write.

Over the weeks of our training, the natural snow line crept lower, the wind began to slice. We hobbled out of the locker room with burned cheeks and spasming quads. By the week of solstice, the sun set on the bus ride home, the Snake River steaming by starlight, my Subaru curving those last miles home in the dark. When I got back to the cabin I would loosen my boots at the door and go straight to the stove to blow on the coals, sliding logs in at an angle, waiting for the cabin to warm enough to take off my down coat.

And so I must have gotten the call somewhere between the resort and home, must have arrived into the orange glow of the cabin already afraid for her, because what I remember is using my rickety college printer to print pixelated pictures of my baby sister—three and a half years younger than I—and taping them to my walls, wiping snot on the sleeves of my jacket as I cried. *My sister could die.* Christine holding our family's new boxer puppy; Christine in her Buffs sweatshirt; all three of us sisters at my college graduation, the previous spring. Just two months earlier I had visited Christine in that dorm room in Colorado, slept on her floor, taken her out for happy hour–priced mac 'n' cheese and pot au chocolat at a fancy Pearl Street restaurant where they served her dessert wine even though she was underage, and we wiggled our eyebrows at each other and didn't say a word. But for much longer than we'd been close, we hadn't been: I was already gone during her high school years, and although we often stayed up late talking when we saw each other, her world then unfolded in a tumble of partying and older guys and emo bands that I, with my unshaven legs and hippie hair and backpacking trips, struggled to relate to. We connected once in a while, but we didn't keep in touch.

That night I cried in the way you do when you understand you have nearly missed something, when you have nearly made a terrible mistake.

The genetic mutation that almost took my sister was one we'd never heard of: congenital long QT syndrome.

If the heart is a muscle, pumping blood by contracting and relaxing, it is also an electrical organ. Each heartbeat unfolds in five separate electrical pulses generated in the sinus node, a patch of tissue in the upper right-hand chamber of the heart, rightfully known as the heart's pacemaker. These electrical pulses crash through the heart like a wave, and to monitor them physicians have labeled each with a letter, P through T. During P, the upper (atrial) chambers act as the little pumps that load the big pumps (the lower chambers of the heart, called ventricles): the right atrium sends oxygen-depleted blood to the right ventricle, and the left atrium sends oxygen-rich blood to the left ventricle. During QRS, the right ventricle pumps out to the lungs for oxygenation, and the left ventricle pumps oxygenated blood out to the body. During the T part of the wave, everything is supposed to electrically reset for the next beat, a process known as repolarization.

If you've ever seen the ziggity-zag of a heartbeat on a monitor in a prime-time hospital drama, you've looked at the PQRST, how it unfolds and unfolds and unfolds as a heart beats onward. An electrocardiogram—or EKG—is the way we capture an image of the heart's electricity, one that allows us to see if electricity is following the right sequence, peaking and dropping in the right places at the right times in the right amount.

We use the same word for hearts and drums; we love a steady beat. A heart is predictable the way the tides are predictable, the way rivers in the desert shrink during the day and expand outward at night.

And yet we cannot take for granted that the heart will ebb and flow at the right time, because sometimes it does not.

In a heart with the type of long QT syndrome my sister has, the physical structure is fine, but repolarization can be prolonged, a problem that becomes exaggerated under certain types of stress. This means the interval from Q to T is—as you might expect from the name—too long. Sometimes when this happens, there are heart cells only half primed at the right moment, so they half fire, triggering other things to half fire. This inconsistency can go unnoticed—a slight palpitation, maybe—or it can cause the rhythm of the heart to spin out of control, unable to pump in the firm, organized manner that gets blood oxygenated and out to the limbs and organs. A heart that quivers instead of pumps fails to get oxygen to the brain.

The lucky faint but wake up when the heart recovers a normal rhythm. The unlucky die of cardiac arrest.

Long QT is most dangerous when you don't know it's there—21 percent of symptomatic patients die within a year if they don't receive treatment. There's a long list of medications to avoid—everything from antihistamines to antimalarials—because they further lengthen the QT interval. Though 90 percent of people with long QT have their first abnormal heart rhythm before age forty, there have been cases of older adults without the genetic mutation who end up with medication-induced long QT syndrome as a side effect of pills they take for other conditions.

There are at least thirteen types of congenital long QT, with three genetic variants accounting for 90 percent of all diagnosed cases. Those with type 1 are most at risk when they exercise, type 3 are most at risk during sleep, and type 2—like my sister—need to avoid being startled. For most types of LQT, taking adrenergic-blocking drugs, known as beta-blockers, can help; these medications decrease the effect of stress hormones in a body, causing the heart to beat more slowly, preventing big spikes in the QT length.

But the heart, sometimes, cannot be controlled. The cardiac defibrillator that my sister had implanted that December was the equivalent of a personal set of emergency-room paddles, a resuscitation device she could carry with her every minute of her life. A small titanium box containing a motherboard, capacitor, and battery, her ICD was connected to her heart by a thin lead wire that ran down her left subclavian vein and screwed into her right ventricle. If she'd had the procedure any later, her surgeon said, she would have received a second wire, screwed into the right atrium, to enable pacing of the heart. These wires contained tiny sensors that could monitor her heartbeat—and if a dangerous arrhythmia were detected, all that quivering instead of pumping, the ICD would shock her heart to disrupt it, delivering between three hundred and eight hundred volts. The heart would flatline. Then, we hoped, the natural rhythm of the heart would kick back in; life would resume.

My mom sent texts when Christine was out of surgery, when she was boarding the plane. In Chicago, my sister spent the month resting. She wore a giant gauze badge over the left side of her chest and followed movement restrictions: *Lift nothing over thirty pounds. Do not raise your arms above shoulder height.* At a Christmas party, her high school friends shied away from the topic of her heart surgery, her cardiac arrests. No one mentioned the square of gauze or the sling she wore to prevent pulling on the incision. Self-conscious, Christine slipped her arm out of her sling now and again; hurting, she slipped it back in. Beneath the gauze, the device settled into the pocket Dr. Oza had carved for it between the pectoral muscle and skin, because there is no natural space in a body for a titanium box. Years later,

Christine told me that she and my mother had huddled together to take off the bandage, audibly gasping with relief when they saw the gentle bump on her chest. "We had no idea what to expect," she said. "We thought it might be huge."

I didn't go home for Christmas that year, working through the holiday rush at the ski mountain, as was required. It was easy not to think about my sister's mortality—the technology had fixed that, right?—and I was busy falling for one of the snowboard instructors, a tall, dangerously charming Hotshot firefighter who came down to my cabin to help split thick rounds of wood, his shirt cast off in a snowbank. It was easy to become absorbed in my life in Wyoming, to ignore what was happening elsewhere, to sneak in ski runs before and after work and stay up late writing angsty love poetry. (That man never did kiss me.) I didn't leave the county for five months.

In the meantime, my family members were slowly filing into doctors' offices to get EKGs, to find out if their QTs were long. My older sister Cindy's was negative. So, too, were my parents', which left the mystery of where the genetic defect came from wide open. They'd call me from their house in Illinois: *Kati, you really need to go in.* I didn't have insurance. *We'll pay for it.* I didn't have the time. I didn't know where to go. Twenty-two-year-olds did not just stop into the hospital for EKGs. *Just call the hospital. It's important.* Whatever, I thought. I was the healthiest person I knew. I taught skiing and rock climbing and ran up mountains. I ate organic food. I lived in the most intact eco-system in the Lower 48—drank fresh snowmelt, inhaled alpine air.

Christine herself said nothing. She was pretending none of this existed.

The first answers came from Texas, in April. One of my dad's older brothers, Chris, went to the doctor for chest pains and was told he had a long QT. Their eldest brother, Steve—a librarian and the de facto family historian—remembered an old story when he heard this. Their grandfather, a railroad engineer known as Pa Choo-Choo, was an only child. Though he'd grown up in a gaggle of half siblings, his mother had died just five months after he was born, when she was twenty. And, as the story went, it was a heart attack.

This was in early March of 1899, three years before the EKG was invented. Heart attacks occur when blood flow to the heart is blocked, by blood clots or clogged arteries, starving the muscle of oxygen and causing parts of it to die. Cardiac arrest, on the other hand, occurs when the electricity of the heart malfunctions and the heart stops effectively pumping blood. But without the knowledge that the heart is a muscular machine driven by current—without the ability to measure the waves of electricity rolling through the body—there would have been no way to distinguish between the two.

One of the diagnostic criteria for long QT syndrome is a history of unexplained young deaths in the family. It seemed like Lena Proctor Standefer, 109 years back, might hold our answer.

One morning in late April of 2008, my sister was on her way to class when she realized she'd forgotten the paper she needed to hand in. Turning, she quickly power walked back to her dorm. As she slid her key card through the reader, an electric current cut her. Before she could think, she was screaming. Had she been electrocuted by the door? Then she knew. She slipped inside the dorm, clutching her chest, and retrieved her paper. Then she headed back to class. Stunned, she stayed the whole period.

At the hospital that afternoon, they told her one of her wires had moved seven millimeters. Unable to read her heart correctly from its new location, the machine had double-counted her heartbeats. It hadn't been a lifesaving shock; it had been a mistake. Until the wire was removed and a new one placed into the appropriate position, her ICD would be a danger to her. And if they turned it off, she would be without her backup.

She was still a freshman in college, facing her second round of finals alongside her second heart surgery. When she went under, her heartbeat was so irregular they had trouble placing the new wire. The surgery went on too long, and this time she woke up, frantically trying to bring her hands to her chest but finding them tied to the bed. "Christine, you have to calm down," Dr. Oza pleaded. She could see the blue sheet draped at her upper chest, knew somewhere down there she was gaping open. "Christine, don't move."

Panic, hot and blue. Then she was out again.

This time there was already a cavern in her body for the metal box, already a yawning red mouth to hold machinery. She got twelve staples and was discharged. She flew home for the summer with my father hauling her suitcase through the airport, her arm in a sling. She'd made it five months into her movement restrictions. A lifelong swimmer and longtime lifeguard with a summer job lined up to coach swimmers and manage the pool, Christine faced another six months out of the water. She was crushed.

CAUSA FINALIS

CHAPTER 2

Jackson, Wyoming
2009

O n the last morning of my first life, I got up early to hike Paint-brush Canyon with a friend. It was a beautiful day after weeks of rain, the trail still sweating off its snow in places, and we took the switchbacks carefully, kicking steps where we needed. Above us, the long gray cliffs of Mount Moran shimmered with runoff, and the fresh smell of dried pine needles, finally uncovered in places, made us feel drunk.

This was June of 2009, and by then I was living in East Jackson with Sam, my boyfriend of a year, in a cabin duplex built to look like a boat: long and narrow, with curved eaves and a boarded-up porthole to the neighbor's side. Our bedroom door was heavy and wood, battened and ledged like the entrance to a captain's quarters. There was a junkyard out front—fenders and flagstone and a rusted VW Beetle with its tires melted into the gravel—and a spot where we stacked our wood. The back of our house was one grand enormous window, and at first we woke every morning to mountains, pink with dawn or ropy with storm clouds. Later, we hung a maroon curtain across so we could make love without the neighbors' kids suddenly trundling into view.

I'd met Sam early in the summer of 2008, when we found our-selves rock climbing with mutual friends at a crag outside Lander, Wyoming. He was a writer and editor, working then for an elite climbing magazine. He sported cute nerdy glasses and grinned with perfect teeth. After a few weeks of his relentless pursuit, on a night we'd been clumsily dancing and drinking Moose Drool together, I let him drive me home from Bluegrass Tuesday to the bed-and-breakfast where I was working for the summer. In those months I slept in an open-air structure we called the Tent Cabin, a building on the side of a hill with no door in the frame and no glass in the windows. "I've got to see this," he said, following me up the steps and through the forest. We lit a row of candles. There in the weeds outside my cabin, we finally kissed by starlight.

He was my first boyfriend. In July, we ditched my narrow army cot in favor of a nest of blankets on the Tent Cabin's wide porch, waking to the shiver of aspen leaves, making love in the open air of the forest. I would try to break up with him briefly three weeks in, under a flickering light in a parking lot near the center of town, folding my arms over my chest as a barrier as he kept trying to kiss me. I'd found myself uncomfortable in the relationship; the evening and morning hours I spent with him used to be my writing hours, and without them I felt unhinged, useless. I counted the ways he didn't fit the image of my dream man: buying cheap hormone-filled meat rather than cuts from local ranchers, playing too much beer pong in the garage with his buddies.

But the day after I tried to break up with him, Sam would run through fields of mud and horseshit at the county fair looking for me, as I sang at a fundraiser with my bluegrass band. He would take me for a long walk under boiling storms, would turn me toward him and burst into tears. "I've been in relationships where the spark's not there, where it's not going to work out," he said, "and this isn't that, Kati."

Three days later, missing him, I agreed to meet him at the fair-grounds. I turned my head away from his kisses. But as we walked among the 4-H rabbits and baby goats, as we babbled together at them, I felt an enormous relief. A tenderness. We went back to his town house that night and tried to make homemade custard-style ice cream, but he fell asleep as I was stirring the dark liquid. Then, decisions: finishing the recipe rather than letting the egg scramble on the heat. Putting the syrup in the fridge. Walking into his room to turn out the light above him. And finally, rather than driving in the immense darkness across the valley, rather than ten miles home, I crawled into his bed. I relented.

The space that opens between two people is never quite predictable, although there are signs, early, of the world they might build. The laughter. The goats. All that first fall, after I moved back south to Hoback at summer's end, I would wake in the low light of my cabin and see Sam on the mattress beside me, clutching to his chest an old bear I kept named Chugach—Chug for short. I had kept Chug around as an adult because he made a great reading pillow. But Sam treated Chug as if he were a being, shyly showing me his own: a sweet scruffy bear with a plaid bow tie named Beary, a soft yellowed lamb—Lambykins—with a pink ribbon at her neck. He dragged a nappy, adorable little white bear in from my car, where it had spent years straddling the gearshift. A red light flashed when you pressed the heart stitched to the bear's chest: Beating Heart Bear.

In October, four months in, Sam told me he loved me while standing on his kitchen table changing a lightbulb. By Christmas, I'd all but stopped making the long drive south to my cabin in Hoback, and shortly after, I moved my things into the big suburban-style house he shared with two friends, initiating our long process of trying to fit two people's clothes in one closet.

But it hadn't been a simple first year. Not long after he told me he loved me—in mid-October of 2008, as the market crashed—the magazine Sam worked for abruptly folded. He got a month's severance. Scrambling to keep himself afloat, he took a job he hated at the local newspaper, filling in as a section editor for someone's maternity leave. All that winter he set his alarm at 3:00 a.m. to make deadline, waking both of us when the moon still hung silver above the snowbanks. Sometimes he fell back asleep and exploded out of bed at 7:00 a.m. like a crazy man. In the morning I stopped by his car at the newspaper and penciled "I love you" onto the icy windshield with my pointer finger.

When we moved to the quirky boat-house in East Jackson that spring, it was our first time just the two of us in a place. The house seemed to hold us in a particular way, both the space and our relationship beautiful and bizarre.

* * *

On the last morning of my first life, I was late getting back from the hike, and due at band practice. I hopped on my bike and coasted the mile from our house to my guitarist's, apologizing as I walked in the door. We had a gig coming up at the Jackson Hole Center for the Arts with other top musicians in the valley, and we'd hardly practiced our pick: the Grateful Dead song "Uncle John's Band," with lyrics I kept getting out of order. We'd barely begun to play when my phone rang.

"Sorry," I said, leaping up, "I have to take this," and my guitarist rolled his eyes at me as I ducked outside into the parking lot to answer the call—from a supervisor at my summer job leading day hikes, whom I'd been waiting to hear from.

Then all I remember is a punch of nausea, and falling.

When I woke the sky was full of swords, clear and sharp, crossing the sky quickly. If I shut my eyes my ears filled with a white sound, roaring, awful. I did not know who or where I was. Finally, the sounds in my ears hissed out, but I couldn't move, couldn't speak, was so nauseated. I waited on my back in the gravel until I was able to croak my guitarist's name, so quiet, then again, a little louder, again and again until finally I heard the guitar slam down and he rushed outside. "Oh my god," he said, and he knelt on the gravel. He tried to help me sit up, and I whimpered, I was so sick, I was so dizzy, I thought I might throw up. He said, "Maybe you got low blood sugar; maybe you're dehydrated," and rushed inside for some fruit juice, tipping it slightly into my mouth.

He called Sam, who had been playing croquet and drinking beer at a yard party a few doors down from our place, and within minutes my blue Subaru was rounding the bend, clattering over the gravel parking lot, and Sam was out, helping me sit up. I moaned; every part of me hurt. I could lift my arm by then and found there was gravel in my forehead, indentations remaining after I brushed it off. I must have fallen face-forward and rolled.

"Let's get you to the hospital," Sam said.

"No," I said. "You can't take me to the hospital. I don't have insurance. If you take me to the hospital now, I will never be able to get insurance again." Sam just looked at me uneasily.

At home, Sam settled me on the couch and went to call my parents. I could hear his low voice in the other room, the murmur of conversation. I knew how he pulled at his hair when he was stressed, and that by the time he came back it would be a tall poof above his forehead.

This was 2009, and the health-care debates were raging. One of the most contentious issues remained the problem of preexisting conditions—an insurer's legal right to refuse to cover medical problems that existed before a person signed up. To buy coverage when you were healthy and get sick on the insurer's watch was the ideal scenario. But insurers weren't going to take on those who were only buying insurance after something had happened—inevitably expensive patients who drained more money than they put into the pool. If those patients got insurance at all, it was without coverage for the care they needed most.

I'd aged off my father's insurance plan when I graduated from college, as was typical then. At the time, this hadn't seemed an injustice. Though my father had helped me with the cost of tuition, he'd also instilled in me the idea that once I graduated, I was responsible for myself. My sisters and I grew up steeped in the mythology of my dad's prudent financial choices—from switching to an in-state school after his freshman year of college to living at home during his first year of law school, then attending night classes for five semesters so that he could work full-time and afford both his apartment and tuition. ("I majored in economics," read a T-shirt he purchased at one point: "To save time, let's just assume I'm always right.") When I chose to pursue my dream of writing as a career after graduation—when I chose to move to the mountains and sagebrush steppes of western Wyoming that I loved—I knew I was shirking the conventional forms of stability he and my mom (an actuarial assistant turned stay-at-home mom turned preschool teacher) had instilled in me. It seemed important that I "do it on my own"—or as "on your own" as you could be if someone else had recently bought you a nice used car and spared you all but a few thousand dollars of college debt, despite your attendance at an expensive liberal arts school a thousand miles from home. The cheap catastrophic insurance plan I purchased that first year didn't enable me to go to the doctor without paying the whole cost of the visit toward my deductible, but I didn't think I would need to see a doctor. I only needed something that could keep me financially solvent in the event I broke my leg skiing.

In my second year out of college, though, I gave up the catastrophic coverage. The economic downturn hit Jackson hard, and I struggled to make enough to pay the premium, several hundred dollars a month. It hadn't occurred to me to ask my parents for the money: I was stubborn, and I was healthy. Most important, as someone who'd always had access to high-quality care through my father's workplace group plans, I didn't understand what could happen without it. The only sick people I knew were old—and covered. I let my insurance plan lapse.

When Sam reappeared in the doorway, his face was hesitant. "I have to take you to the hospital," he said. "I'm sorry; I have to."

"Okay," I said quietly.

For even then, of course, I knew where this was going. Since the moment I'd sat up in the parking lot, I could feel fate pulling at me, a deep magnetic current that was sweeping me off somewhere.

In my narrow bed in the emergency room at St. John's Medical Center, with Sam still in the waiting room, I told the physician my sister had long QT syndrome, that he should check my QT. The doctor ordered my first EKG, disappeared while they covered me in sticky electrodes, and came back without fanfare. "Well, yes," he said. "You do have an abnormally long QT interval, so it looks like you have it," he said.

A wail erupted from my body, so loud and aggrieved I almost couldn't recognize it as my own. The sound of what my life was about to become.

"Oh," he said nervously, leaning forward to awkwardly pat my shoulder, "now don't do that." The grieving itself, he insinuated, put me at a higher risk of cardiac arrest.

But heart, I had no alternative for grief.

* * *

Later, doctors would ask if I'd had symptoms, and I would say no. A QT interval can be long without deteriorating into arrhythmia; a long QT is not necessarily something you can feel.

But the truth was a matter of interpretation, a question of what should be linked to what. One night that winter I'd woken gasping for air, something I would later learn is a common cardiac symptom. I'd battled upper-chest anxiety for months, which I ascribed to food sensitivities—running seven-week elimination diets—but which could have been palpitations. And one afternoon, sprinting on the treadmill at the climbing gym, my heart had suddenly started beating out of my body, a hammering sensation far beyond my pace that terrified me. I hit the red emergency Stop button and sat quickly at the end of the belt.

Whatever it was ceased. I took a few deep breaths. Bodies, I knew, sometimes did weird things for no particular reason. I got up, restarted the treadmill, slowly began gaining speed. But when I felt my heart suddenly accelerate again, I slammed the Stop button and stepped away from the machine, too scared to continue.

Somehow none of this struck me as notable; each instance slid away without remark. Despite my mother's periodic demands that I have an EKG done, my sister's story remained remote to me. In the rare instances I'd seen Christine since my move to that valley, she hadn't told me much about her experience—focusing, instead, on her work at a noodle restaurant, her on-again, off-again long-distance boyfriend, the upcoming events at her sorority. Her scar was easily covered by her shirt.

Some part of me, I can admit now, beat a wide path around having that EKG. If I were diagnosed with long QT syndrome, I knew my life as I had fashioned it would be over. I was a ski instructor and climbing guide who lived alone in areas without cell service, who needed to evacuate clients from the backcountry, who loved to wander in solitude off trail. Casually walking into a hospital and paying cash for a test could upend my world, so I didn't.

But some part of me knew: if anyone else had it, it would be me.

* * *

The hospital kept me overnight for observation and in the morning released me with a prescription for beta-blockers and a Monday appointment to see the cardiologist down in Salt Lake City, our closest option—a five-hour drive. Because I'd recently lost consciousness and hadn't been on the medication long, I wasn't allowed to drive, so my father began pricing plane tickets for me. We had family friends in Salt Lake, he mused; maybe they could take me to my appointment.

"Lady," Sam said when I told him. "Of course I'll take you."

"But you have to work," I said.

He just looked at me.

For the next two days Sam did not leave my side. A mania swept into our bodies, the energy overripe and frantic. How were we to live if at any moment I could die? We felt we should be *doing something* about this, except there was nothing to *do*. There was only going through the motions of living: doing the laundry, cooking meals, hypervigilant about every sensation in my body. There was only this in-between space: no answers yet about whether, like Christine, I would need an ICD, no answers yet about whether I could continue working in the backcountry, no answers yet about what that emergency room bill would total when it came roaring into my mailbox.

On Sunday, Sam's twenty-seventh birthday, we drove through Idaho in ricocheting storms, the sky luminous and orange with sunset as far as we could see. Roofs beside the interstate glimmered silver, tall grass bent green with the wind. We ate handfuls of soft tacos from a drive-through and got sick, too used to our summer farm share, and all the way Sam held my hand, protective.

We arrived into the silence of the city at midnight, slept at the family friend's, and got up early to go to the clinic. Salt Lake was an inferno, all blazing heat and glinting metal and concrete, the traffic creeping toward downtown. Finally we reached the right high-rise, took the elevator, and settled into the waiting room, a place with cream walls and composite carpet. The room was filled with the elderly and their adult children, who pushed them in wheelchairs, who brought their clipboards back to the seating area for them. For the first time I felt the strange experience of having all eyes on me, of being the youngest one in a cardiology office: *What are you here for?*

No one had told me about the treadmill test, and after they took me back and affixed all the sticky electrodes I was becoming used to, I found myself walking, then running, in my pair of sporty Mary Janes, my breasts flopping around without a sports bra. The technician tried to find my maximum heart rate. She cranked up the incline, then sped up the machine; we went in intervals until her eyes widened. "Tell us when you get too tired to continue!" she said, aghast.

"Of course, you are a bit younger than most of our patients," her partner said from the corner, tracking my vitals. They were looking for how much my heart could manage, what it looked like at maximum, whether there were any "plumbing" problems—issues with the physical heart—or just the electrical irregularity of long QT. Finally, without having maxed out my fitness ability, we all just got tired of the test, and they hustled me to an ultrasound table so they could watch my heart pump, sliding the cold, lubed-up knob beneath my breast. There it was, wild with movement on the screen, multicolored and beating.

"Your heart is beautiful," the technician said, beaming at me, like it was a pregnancy, some kind of new life. *My heart.*

I would learn over the years that it's not a cardiology visit without a long wait in a freezing room, and that time was no different. The man who finally emerged to speak to me was fleshy and of medium height, wearing glasses. He quickly told me, looking at my numbers, that I did not need a defibrillator. As long as I took the beta-blockers they'd prescribed, he said, I would be fine.

"I feel like we've been a little over the top in our precautions," I told him, "so I thought I would ask: What, exactly, do I need to be afraid of?"

"Basically everything," he said. He thought for a moment. "You should probably never swim again." I stared at him. After a moment he added, "Light tennis and golf would probably be okay."

With this, the visit was over.

* * *

In that tower above the sweltering city, my life ground to a halt. For the first time rage, instead of fear, welled up in my body. The doctor had ignored my age, my explanation of my life. He had simultaneously told me that I was fine—that there was no need to implant a defibrillator, that the pills would do their work—and that I would be in danger at all times. He had told me that what I loved best about being alive, including the way I made my living, was to be off-limits, and he had done so quickly, casually, without meeting my eyes, as though this would come without loss. I could not, in that short meeting, tell him of the first morning I'd woken in Wyoming's backcountry, the summer I was fifteen; how I'd slept out under the stars on a tarp in a valley ringed with pines and heartleaf arnica, and how in the morning I'd stirred to a roar that sounded precisely like a highway. I'd lain there for many minutes, the dew on my sleeping bag slightly frozen, trying to figure out, after our long drive down, after the washboard roads and a five-mile hike, what road could possibly be nearby.

It was only then that I recognized the sound of the wind.

How was a person to live if she were simultaneously fine and in danger at every moment? In the weeks that followed, I spent hours on the phone with Sam's friends who were doctors, trying to understand. I connected with an organization called the Sudden Arrhythmia Death Syndromes Foundation—SADS—and their staff spent whole afternoons thinking through my situation, trying to pin down what we did and didn't know about long QT syndrome and how it related to exercise. From what I could parse, physical exertion itself is rarely dangerous for those of us with type 2 (exercise is type 1's trigger), yet many type 2 kids are diagnosed and yanked from their sports teams as a precaution. That type 2's QT interval lengthens based on an adrenaline response means that certain parts of physical activity might be more dangerous than others—the burst of a sprint, the surprise of someone coming from behind for the ball. But beneath all my questions lay a bare medical answer: no one knew yet. In 2009, we didn't yet have longitudinal studies examining how people's activity levels translated to cardiac events. Long QT syndrome is believed to be rare, affecting about one in seven thousand people, although it is thought that many remain undiagnosed. According to the National Heart, Lung, and Blood Institute, as many as three to four thousand children and young adults die every year of long QT syndrome. Organizations such as SADS work to get out in front of this—helping people recognize warning faints, supporting efforts to place automatic external defibrillators (AEDs) beside playing fields, encouraging the screening of young athletes using EKGs, and creating a pool of people who could turn to each other for help—but there was a long way to go. No one could give me an answer.

To take groups hiking into the backcountry, it went without saying, was unacceptable: whether or not the physical exercise put me at risk, I would be miles from the nearest medical facility if, say, I were startled by a bear, the kind of thing that happened from time to time in this line of work. But I would lead the groups anyway, as my life folded in on me, for I had bills to pay. The groups I was slated to lead that summer weren't backpacking, I rationalized. We would never be, say, thirty miles from a trailhead, hauling pots and tents toward some high tarn. My clients stayed in high-end hotels in town and ate at restaurants with elk heads mounted to the walls. During our hikes my co-leader and I carried only first aid kits, tablecloths, chicken salad, and fresh chocolate chip cookies on our backs.

Yet we did drive to remote trailheads up on the Divide, hike ten miles at a stretch, tackle steep paths red with mud. I had been doing this work long enough to know that we managed risk every time we went out.

The beta-blockers, once they built up in my system, left me dizzy and short of breath, keeping my heart rate artificially low even when my body needed more oxygen. As I hiked in front of my clients, I was often close to passing out, watching my edge. I tried to stay fast enough to be professional, to keep a lead on those knobby-kneed old men in beige jungle shirts who'd spent their retirements doing nothing but hiking—but I was always scared. I never knew if the sensations I felt in my chest were the heart condition itself or the medication, was never sure if I was in danger. As we hiked deep into the forest, I swallowed down anger as my clients—mostly older and wealthy, often conservative—weighed in on the health-care debates, usually on the side of politicians whose plans would have left me without care for the foreseeable future.

And so death stalked me for the first time that summer, arriving with its hot breath on the back of my neck. I went running out on the National Elk Refuge road and found myself sitting at its edge, spinning, looking out at the long dry grasses that gleamed with silver in the wind. I woke in the morning with death sitting heavy on my chest, a fatigue clotting my eyes, and could not forget it. One day I had to call Sam from a strip of grass not far from the library, where I'd hopped off my bike, dizzy and palpitating, afraid I'd topple forward into traffic. He loaded the bike into his Jeep with the sort of sad silence that I have come to know as a part of illness in general, but especially for those who are young and sick—those from whom something is being taken that they did not yet realize they had. What gave me pleasure in life was hopping on my bike to streak downtown; what managed my moods was intense exercise; what made me feel *me* was to move through the wild. I didn't understand, actually, what the alternative to doing these things was; I saw a life full of nothing. I saw a person who wasn't me.

I kept thinking: my sister almost died in bed all those times. However much I might twist my life into one of caution and stillness, avoiding everything, it could be someone's ringing cell phone, the siren of a passing ambulance. I hadn't been hiking in the backcountry when I passed out in that parking lot. I had taken a call. If death wanted to find me, there was no stopping it. Maybe in this the Salt Lake cardiologist was right: nothing was safe.

Sam had been my first sex partner, at age twenty-three, after many years of wishing for love and being stubborn enough to turn down sex without it. Late those nights, I would slide on top of him as I always had, but find myself all but passing out, the beta-blockers capping my heart rate at the moments I needed it to quicken most. In those moments I found myself in a silent, angry bargaining: I would, in an instant, have traded safety for danger in order to stay in those sharp, flushed moments where illness had no right to intrude.

"I'm only motherfucking twenty-four," I said to Sam one night, lying frustrated on my back, trying to deep-breathe my way back into my body, his chest glistening with the sweat of *almost*.

"Maybe they could lower the dose?" he said. "If you would still be safe?"

So when my father suggested I see my sister's electrophysiologist in Boulder for a second opinion, and when he offered to buy the plane ticket—to make sure I didn't need a defibrillator and to make sure I was on the right dose of the drug—I said yes.

Dr. Oza was a small, very intense man with glasses and neatly combed black hair who'd gone to medical school in India before completing his internship, residency, and cardiology fellowships in the United States. He carefully documented my complaints of extreme fatigue, the sexual dysfunction. He told me the way they make decisions about long QT treatment is to assign points for certain attributes, then tally them up. Points for family history of sudden death. Points for biological sex, since androgen is a protective factor in males (they're most at risk before puberty) and females are most likely to die suddenly during menstruation or just after giving birth. Points for documented syncopes and torsades de pointes waves. Points for the length of your uncorrected QT interval. A QT interval considered normal is usually below 440 milliseconds; mine, at intake in Jackson, was 520 ms, and during my treadmill test in Utah it had rocketed to 580 ms, even though I'd started my beta-blocker prescription just a few days earlier.

To have a long QT interval is not a problem one would likely notice or feel. But the increased repolarization time can lead to the heart's getting out of sync, which in turn can lead to anything from minor palpitations to cardiac arrest and sudden cardiac death.

"I know the doctor in Salt Lake suggested that you would be fine on beta-blockers for the rest of your life," Dr. Oza said. "But given your family history, I strongly recommend you have an ICD implanted."

I blinked back tears. "I have to think about it," I said. The thought of having a computer placed in my body panicked me. Not the scar I would carry on the left side of my chest or even the surgery, exactly; it was the idea of becoming a technological person. It was the idea that a human was a series of systems, and any one of them might be replaced by technology, that my human problems would now be tech problems. This was 2009, and while Sam had stood in line for his first iPhone in Salt Lake City after my appointment, I still carried a flip phone from 2004. I was by nature resistant to electronics. I didn't watch TV or play video games, and lived vaguely angry about the idea of upgrades, the way companies push you along unnecessarily, rendering what worked perfectly fine suddenly unusable because of leapfrogging changes in hardware and software.

And I was not, as so many still were then, disconnected from the resources it took to make an object. During college I'd been the co-chair of the environmental club on campus, a role that fell to me naturally after Bush-era natural gas leasing threatened the Wyoming Range—those same scrappy mountains where I'd come into myself—sending me into a panic. In an environmental justice class, I'd visited a molybdenum mine in Questa, New Mexico, which had reopened in the wake of September 11, after the declaration of war. Before our visit to Questa, I'd never thought about the fact that military operations required steel, and lots of it—tanks, planes, Humvees—and that steel required alloys like molybdenum. That to make basically anything required earth. That the wartime boom economy rested on the backs of mountains. Here were the details about Questa that were hard to shake: the hair of the children turned white. Their fingernails streaked white. White blobs poured from the faucets. Dried tailings whipped into dust clouds that blinded the valley. Eyes and throats burned. The dried-up and bleached carcasses of cattle appeared on lawns. Following spill after spill, the Red River was declared dead. In Questa, I learned for the first time how many things could go wrong: pipes ruptured, tailings flooded the river, heavy metals leached into the groundwater. Yet many in the town cheered the mine's return: what made the town sick was also what paid its residents. The mine had reopened to capture flush contracts sliding downstream from the Department of Defense, but the ore would also go toward wheelchairs and mountain bikes. And so I carried with me a visceral sense of the complications of living in an industrial society. No object materialized without impacts. No technology—no matter its benefits—existed without stakes.

I couldn't in that visit articulate to Dr. Oza—or anyone else, really—what my reservations were about the defibrillator. To argue against a lifesaving technology when it was your own life to save sounded ridiculous. But I carried a deep unease; I needed more time. I didn't know you could simultaneously desire and resist something so strongly. I only knew that to place microelectronics above my breast, to hold circuitry in my very body, to become a soul bearing software, seemed an action in opposition to so many of the things I loved most.

"In the meantime, I'm not comfortable with you spending time in the backcountry," Dr. Oza was saying. "No rock climbing. Light exertion only." My head swam.

And then, instead of decreasing the medication, he increased it, from forty milligrams per day to sixty. The message was loud and clear: you are in danger. "What are your concerns about implantation?" he said.

"I'm uninsured," I said. "So I don't know how that could even be an option."

"Well," Dr. Oza said, "if you get your surgery at Boulder Community Hospital, I will donate my fee."

"I just don't know," I said. "Are you sure I need it?"

Dr. Oza peered at me, as though reconsidering. "Has anyone ever told you that you have an arrhythmia?" he said.

"No," I said. Then: "Actually, yes— one of the nurses at St. John's mentioned that I'd had a very scary arrhythmia the night they kept me over after the syncope. In the middle of the night."

"Okay," he said. "That wasn't in the records they sent me. I need you to go back to them and ask them for *everything*. Tell them I want the whole file. Have them send it to me by fax if they want." He looked at me squarely. "Your case is on the edge. It's not clear. We can't confirm that you experienced cardiac arrest. But based on your family history and the length of your QT interval, I think you would be much safer if you had the device. It's important to know what's on those overnight strips."

On the rainy morning Dr. Oza called about my records, my house was full of Sam's cousins. By then it was early August, and the four of them—all hobbit-size and sporting the same button nose—were about to head up the Grand Teton. They were busy dividing gear, distributing Clif Bars, and rolling rain jackets into the outside pockets of their packs while I was hiding in bed, watching the gray storm clouds roil in our skylight.

Then Dr. Oza's nurse Emily called. "Kati?" she said. "Dr. Oza received your records, and he's had a chance to review them, and he'd like to speak with you about them. Do you have a minute?"

Yes, I did.

When I hung up, I was in tears. I sat on the edge of our red comforter, the curtains drawn back, watching the water splatter against the glass of our big window, with the muffled sounds of the boys cooking eggs coming through the heavy wood door. Dr. Oza had pored through the stacks of EKGs from the night I spent hooked up at the hospital, he said, and he'd discovered strips showing the torsades de pointes morphology in the early morning hours. Meaning "twisting of the points," the term refers to the arrhythmia specifically associated with long QT. The EKGs mapped out on paper what it looked like for a heart to quiver instead of beat.

"The strips were very disturbing," he told me. "You would have one or two normal beats, followed by four beats of torsades. Then three normal beats, five torsades—two normal beats, a few more torsades." For several minutes, he said, I hung on the line between rhythm and arrhythmia. I could have so easily spun out of control.

Dr. Oza paused. "You need to make your arrangements," he said.

When Sam poked his head back in, he saw me crying. "I have to have the surgery," I told him, and he folded me into his arms. We stood silently, with the boys making a racket on the other side of the door and the rain sliding over the house, both of us so scared.

In the final weeks of summer, when the elk were beginning to move secretly and steadily in the forests toward their winter ground, my parents flew in from their home, outside Chicago. It was the first time we'd seen each other since I passed out in June. They stayed at a bed-and-breakfast near the center of Jackson, a beautiful wooden house bursting with baskets of geraniums. Sam and I rode our bikes downtown to meet them for coffee. We ate curly fries and danced at Bluegrass Tuesday at the Wort Hotel, hiked Jackson Peak, and canoed across String Lake on a brilliantly sunny day. We biked Antelope Flats Road across the valley in a fine mist, waiting quietly on the side of the road for groups of bison to disperse, and when I pulled over halfway up Kelly Hill, my head spinning, my throat tight, my dad called out in his red raincoat: "What's the matter? You get beta-blocked?"

I nodded. "I'm okay," I said, and we waited until it passed.

On their last night in town, we convened in the red-walled, book-lined library of the bed-and-breakfast. My father, tall and brown-haired, wore circular glasses that made him look like the intellectual he was. My mother, with bangs and blond hair to her shoulders, always tan despite her religious use of sunscreen, filled a napkin with cookies. The elephant in the room all trip, of course, had been the question of how I might access surgery. Though they'd wanted to meet with just me, Sam was adamant. "Of course I want to be there!" he said, and we were all secretly pleased.

Over white teacups of decaf coffee, we reviewed my options. Could I get on Medicaid to pay for the surgery? No. In 2009, you had to fit certain categories to qualify—like being blind or being a parent to a young child. My dismal income alone didn't qualify me. Some states had a Medicaid expansion program that kicked in if you accrued a certain amount of medical debt, but Wyoming wasn't one of them. Some states had high-risk insurance pools, which cost a lot to buy into but would cover you after a waiting period. Wyoming wasn't one of these, either. Our little hospital in Jackson, St. John's, had provided financial aid for my emergency-room visit. But they were too small to offer advanced cardiac care, and I'd already confirmed that you couldn't somehow transfer your local status to the nearest hospital that did.

"Kati, is there a possibility of finding a job in Jackson with benefits?" my dad said.

"I applied for that social work job," I said. But we all knew that in overeducated Jackson, with the economy plummeting, my qualifications did not translate to a professional job with the state.

I was beginning to understand there was not going to be a way to salvage the life I'd been living. The life I had known was gone, unrecoverable, not durable enough to weather this health crisis. In the past two years, I had taught writing and skiing and backpacking, sung at weddings and circled fancy parties offering hors d'oeuvres. I had swept cabins and figure-modeled, scrubbed toilets and made beds, run birthday parties and written grants. I thought, in my own way, I was doing it: finding a way to stay in the valley, publishing some poems, working on a novel. But I had failed myself in some other way, I saw then, in the precariousness of being spottily employed, in not keeping insurance, in trying to prioritize a writing life. I wished desperately, for my parents' sake, to be some other version of myself: studying international relations or law, coordinating programs or teaching somewhere, taking a salary and insurance from a university or think tank or nonprofit.

I had been authentic to my deepest desires at the cost of my own security—and this seemed fine until it was security I needed. Yet in truth I couldn't imagine living another way, without attention to what made me come alive, without prioritizing the craft that felt like my purpose on the planet. It would take years for me to understand that I had not failed myself as much as been failed by a health-care system that required a particular submission to conventionality—a positioning some couldn't access at all, and which required that the rest of us remain smaller, less bold and creative in our living, more attached to institutions of power. I was born for muddy, ragged places, and time that moved according to a different logic, and now despair rose in me, for the conventional routes to insurance felt far away and impossible—and, more than anything, built for someone else.

An old professor of mine, whom I'd asked for advice, had suggested I seek heart surgery abroad. He'd said there were lots of safe countries where a procedure could be done more cheaply. The suggestion fell flat, my parents dismissive.

Dr. Oza's nurse Emily had warned me that the surgery could cost as much as $180,000 without insurance because of the way uninsured patients didn't benefit from the negotiated-down rates insurance companies received. Why didn't I have the surgery and then declare bankruptcy? I didn't have much to lose: a beat-up Subaru and a bunch of old backpacking gear. Even my skis were ten years old. But my dad widened his eyes, shook his head. "Let's avoid that if at all possible," he said.

"Could you be someone's political darling?" my mom asked.

"Yeah, maybe if you could make one of the senators associated with health-care reform aware of you, they could raise some publicity and money," my dad said.

"Too bad Wyoming representatives aren't the ones making the case for reform," Sam said. "I don't know who we would approach for that."

We were hitting a wall, and just one more idea sat heavy between us. My dad spoke it out loud. "But in Colorado Oza would donate his surgical fee, and if you wait long enough to establish residency, there's a program that might help with your other costs?"

"Yes," I said. "The Colorado Indigent Care Program. Dr. Oza's nurse was telling me about it. And I heard from one of my Colorado friends that it saved her from crazy bills after she tore her ACL. But you have to really live there. Or they have to think you do." I paused. "I looked it up. Residency means three months, or as soon as you're employed." Sam squeezed my hand. "I could go, become a resident, have the surgery, and come home again."

My dad fixed his gaze on me. "How soon could you move?"

I swallowed. "I'm figure-modeling Monday and Wednesday. It's $30 an hour, all day, so it's worth staying for."

"So the first week of September?" My mom nodded.

"Listen, Kati," my dad said, leaning forward. "I can't pay for the surgery. That would be financially ruinous." He was speaking as someone who'd just taken a hit in the recession, who'd spent years working for one corporation that filed for bankruptcy and then another that seemed always to be announcing layoffs, who'd just paid for one daughter's college and was on to the next. Someone who'd suddenly been saddled with the moral hazard of his daughter's passions.

"But I'm not going to let you go under," he said, and my eyes filled with tears. "I will help you," he said. "Until you get a job. With rent and food. I'm not going to get involved with things like your student loans. I would guess that you can go a few months without paying them with only minor penalty, and you may be able to defer. That will be your deal. Let's just communicate about what you need."

"Thank you," I said. What he offered filled me with both shame and relief.

"It's only few months," my dad said.

"Yeah." I looked at Sam. "It's only a few months."

But it didn't feel like a few months. I knew how slippery life could be, the way we end up in places we didn't mean—how when you opened a door and walked through it, sometimes it shut behind you. As I looked at job listings and apartment listings in Boulder over the week that followed, a deep grief pulled at me. I'd moved to Wyoming thinking I would build my life there. I'd first come to that valley as a fourteen-year-old and had missed only two summers since. I'd written two senior theses on the area. This had been the place that opened me, that brought me to myself. Spending my summers in the heady, hot smell of sage, ducking moose in the willows. Judging autumn by the moment the fireweed bloomed its top raceme. At the edge of winter pulling the bird feeders inside, so the bears wouldn't come onto the roof for them; feeding the fire on those coldest winter nights, walking out the back door into forest that went on for hundreds of miles, snowshoeing across valleys where the only marks in the snow revealed the drama of a fox chasing lunch. A great many people came to that valley and moved on without thrusting roots into its rocky soil, but this was not my story.

Yet I knew that the sooner I went, the sooner I would become a Colorado resident. The sooner I could have the surgery. The sooner I could move on with my life. The defibrillator, though I loathed the thought of it, was the answer to the threat of death.

I could not live, I was realizing, without that answer.

Six days before I drove to Boulder, Christine used her cell phone alarm to wake up instead of the special alarm she had been using since her diagnosis, which slowly raised its volume to prevent startling. Before she was fully conscious, she felt her heart beating out of her chest, bold terrible thumps. Then a strange vision: our childhood dog skidding, sliding unstoppably into the kitchen island—

CRACK.

The sound of a voice screaming. Her own.

The e-mail she sent had the subject line "the reason for my defib." Attached was a printout from the St. Jude Medical device interrogation. *Diagnosis: Ventricular Fibrillation. Time to diagnosis. 3.75 seconds. Cycle Length: 240 milliseconds/250 beats per minute. Therapy: 36 joules/830 volts. Episode duration: 20 seconds.*

The torsades de pointes images, terrible and jagged, without rhythm, a monster's teeth, interrupted on the printout by a tiny lightning bolt. A flatline. Then the heart's resumed beating.

By then she had been shocked four times: The first, when her wire moved. The second, in the fall of 2008, while running with a friend— and there was no evidence of arrhythmia, just the defibrillator's thresholds set too low. The third, earlier that summer, had also been unnecessary: her heart rate elevated from exertion during a lifeguard competition, the heartbeat only slightly irregular.

This fourth time, the shock saved her life.

On Thursday it happened again, she wrote in her journal. *It was the real deal.* Torsades de pointes. *The defib went off and saved my life. Now it's not such a pain in the ass. Now it's scary.* She wanted to talk to her long-distance boyfriend, but it was late, and she was tired, and if the phone rung while she was sleeping, she could go into cardiac arrest again. She would have to turn off her phone.

What if it happens again? I know it works. I know I'll be okay. But the unknown, the fact that it happens at all. The fact that I have a lethal heart condition. One day, it will kill me.

On my last weekend in town, Sam and I took his little sailboat up to Slide Lake, where he'd been teaching me, over the last year, to harness the wind. I could tack back and forth. I could duck the boom. Most important, I could hold Sam's can of beer while he steered. He looked beautiful that day, his blue eyes catching the sun, his beard the perfect length and glinting just the slightest bit auburn. From time to time he leaned forward to kiss me, and I could feel myself grieving already: for these dry buttes, for a boat on a lake, for the man grinning back.

"You should probably never swim again," I said in my best cardiologist voice, my lips puckered. Sam rapped his knuckles against my life vest.

"You just keep this on, lady," he said.

That night we stayed in a nearby campground with a friend and her sweet dog. I couldn't shake the feeling that this was the last time. Our fire seemed extravagant. We sliced local bison steaks and vegetables into foil packets and pushed them into the coals with a big stick. I stayed out late writing, where I could hear Sam's soft breathing through the tent fabric, where he lay clutching my teddy bear. I was separating, splitting, and one of me was staying there in Jackson, continuing to live the life I'd worked toward; the other would go stumbling forward blindly, into a life she did not want, a life she did not mean to have, a life she kept insisting could not be—would absolutely not be—good.

It was the relief of continuing to be alive at all that drove me out of the place I most loved.

Midmorning on September second, Sam and I stood at the edge of our long gravel drive, at our boat-cabin, holding each other as I sobbed.

"How do I keep you?" he asked, stricken.

The last thing I saw of East Simpson Avenue, driving away, was my love in the side mirror, breaking into a dead run. He chased the car until I crossed Redmond, his shirt a maroon blur. Then his feet seemed to slap against the black pavement, his body lurching as he tried to stop following, momentum carrying him farther than he meant to go.

Then I was alone, turning down familiar drives. Taking the back route through town by habit, to avoid the tourists and strip malls. Passing the fairgrounds where Sam and I got back together after that very brief breakup. I bridged the Snake River, turned left at Hoback Junction, and passed my beloved ranch, my old cabin in the pines, all the way crying *goodbye, goodbye.*

Even in those first days of September, the silver sheen of autumn had dropped over the land. The red willows along the Hoback River pierced me. The damp, high canyon walls. The river itself, pale, icy, throwing up ribbons of whitewater as it bounced over rocks. The hills had already begun to blanch, yellow, and the air was slightly smoky with the residue of another round of forest fires. I cried all the way to Rock Springs.

Then the great span of the plains stretched before me.

On my first afternoon in Boulder, my sister took me to Half Fast Subs when she got out of class. At the front door, she pushed a few dollars into my hand. "Get a pitcher of Long Islands," Christine said, then went outside to save a table.

On the patio, sunglassed and underage, she poured for us. We sat on the wood slats at dusk, and for the first time I touched the smooth line of her scar, the hard spot above her left breast. I realized she'd never told me about her surgery, a year and a half earlier, and I looked her in the eye. "What will it be like?"

She looked away. "The doctors tell you nothing," she said. And then she told me herself. How riding in cars would be torture, the seat belt pressing onto the incision, and the defibrillator—not yet held in place by scar tissue—bumping up and down inside the body cavity. How I would have to go to salons to have my hair washed in those lean-back sinks so I didn't get the stitches wet or, on the other hand, force the weight of the device against the stitches from the inside, by leaning forward. How I would not be able to dress myself or do the dishes or carry anything or sit up or lie down or reach up. How my friends might be awkward. And the ache would be deep and awful.

She cried, and I cried, and as the night darkened and traffic rolled up and down Broadway, people pushed in beside us, took over our table, until finally we were just two drunk sisters leaning in together in the midst of a party, except for the strange, tender way we kept touching the upper left quadrant of our chests.

CAUSA EFFICIENS

CHAPTER 3

Sylmar, California
2013

"Can you see it breathing?" Roy Boehner said. The two of us stood shoulder to shoulder, leaning forward, slightly hunched, as though we were peering through the clear window of a hospital nursery. Except the scuffed yellow glass formed the front of a welding machine that laser-sealed defibrillators, and what breathed in front of us was a blue rubber glove.

On the day I made it to St. Jude Medical's Sylmar manufacturing facility, half an hour outside LA, it had been ten months since I took those accidental shocks on a soccer field in Tucson. They were months in which I'd never quite lost the scorched sensation beneath my breastbone, months in which I'd never regained trust in my ICD. Into that hollow burrowed the strange question that had arisen, as though from nowhere, as I lay on my back that night: What did I carry inside me?

That I had metal in my body was so obvious as to be absurd. That this metal had an origin—that it had been tugged from the insides of mountains—descended on me like a long-buried memory, which, once surfaced, could not be pushed under again. In the weeks after the shocks—terrified lightning could strike at any moment, from an open sky—I found myself drawn to the internet, to St. Jude Medical's patient hotline, to try to understand the contents of a defibrillator, my parts and pieces. For in the three years the ICD had been in my body, my cells had regenerated, my skin and stomach. The device had become one of the oldest parts of me, more me than me. Its fingers had grown into my heart, its surface covered in waves of clots; my tissues reached out to hold it. And yet the way it felt inside me after the shocks was different: as though violence lay embedded in the metal itself. As though inside my body lived an entire history of loss.

What the patient line would tell me I wrote down in lists. Much of it, they said, was a trade secret. And so I emailed consultants I found online, asking them to list out the likely minerals in the device. I read the press releases that announced St. Jude's contracts, I emailed their employees, I looked up their filings with the Securities and Exchange Commission, trying to determine where the metal came from. In those early days I wanted most to know whether I carried "conflict minerals" inside my breast—defined in this case as tin, tantalum, tungsten, and gold from hand-dug pits in the eastern provinces of the Democratic Republic of the Congo, where armed groups used debt bondage, extortion, and extralegal taxation to profit from the global demand for consumer electronics, terrorizing local populations with the weapons they bought through the sale of this high-priced rock. In Tucson, under the dim light of my bedside lamp, I lay curled in bed with books about the DRC and its long history of conflict, detailing long lists of the acronyms of armies and militias, keeping my window cracked for the crisp creosote smell of a desert winter rain.

I cared about conflict minerals because of a class I'd taken during college in which we traveled to the West African nation of Sierra Leone, one of several countries where the uncut minerals known as blood diamonds bankrolled a series of rebel wars in the 1990s. There, armed groups took control of the diamond-producing areas in the west of the country and forced those they captured to pan for stones in soupy rivers, using the sales to buy weapons and drugs. Though the class was focused on the questions of postwar aid and development, it was impossible not to become intimate with the war itself. Burned cars still lined the highway. Bullet holes studded old rebel checkpoints. We met a woman forced to be the "wife" of a rebel commander, whose real husband refused to take her back after the war. On Aberdeen Beach, a man my own age softly told me he was a Lost Boy—a former child soldier, taken at age seven on his way to school. Day by day, the term *conflict minerals* became visceral to me: how a hand-dug mine became an engine of devastation. If we accept that some forms of human conflict are inevitable, the question of what that conflict looks like—and how long it goes on—depends in part on financing.

But attempting to pin down whether conflict minerals from the DRC might be in my body opened more questions than it answered. "Trade secrets," it dawned on me, might actually mean something more like, *No patient has ever asked us before.* All companies publicly listed on the U.S. stock exchanges had recently been required to begin the long, complicated process of determining whether tin, tantalum, tungsten, or gold from the eastern DRC or surrounding areas were used in their products—the consequence of new legislation—but these results wouldn't be available for years yet. And although the story of conflict minerals offered a particularly dramatic illustration of what it might take to save a life like my own or my sister's, it occurred to me that not forcing labor in a mine or buying weapons with the revenue was perhaps the least we could ask for. Conflict minerals formed the far end of a spectrum, and I didn't know what the rest of that spectrum looked like. A simple yes or no could not tell me what I sought, which was how my body was linked to others'. There was some calculation I was seeking, a slippery balance, the proportions by which the object inside me had improved or destroyed along the way. In this I realized I was thinking as much of nonhumans as humans, for to mine was to rummage inside the earth, and there were ways to do this that seemed reasonable and ways that weren't at all. What I wanted was to see the other humans along the supply chain; what I wanted was to touch the mountain. The thought flickered, then caught as a flame: I wanted to know whether the thing in my body was worth making. That my life was worth what it took.

The Sylmar facility—located in LA's North Valley, not far from where the 405 twists into Interstate 5—was the place I'd come to begin my long backward reach into the supply chain. There were many things I could not know about the origins of the device, but this was not one of them: the titanium box that lay above my left breast had been in these rooms.

The glove reached its fingers toward us, each one perfectly erect. Then it shrank back. Then reached. "That's the helium," Roy said. Using helium during the welding process, he told me, keeps the metal on defibrillators from oxidizing. Roy smiled, rubbing one of his graying temples. He was my tour guide for the day: a bulky man in a button-down shirt and pin-striped pants, with a smooth, almost overaccommodating voice. He'd met me in the lobby, where a wall-mounted monitor flashed my (misspelled) name: V.I.P. status.

"You can touch it," he said, nodding at the glove, but I only poked it carefully with the tip of one index finger. It bobbled.

Inside the glass, a metal clamp held two titanium half shells already fitted with microelectronics, a capacitor, and a battery—a defibrillator waiting to be sealed. When the assembly line ran, an employee put her hands into the gloves, made sure everything was lined up, and sent the computer the okay.

The computer then generated a laser, which heated the device from twenty-one degrees Celsius to more than 1,400 degrees. A metal arm rotated the device, and in ninety seconds *parts* became *thing*. Nickel silver copper cobalt gold tantalum tin. The defibrillator was sealed.

This moment, more than any other, signaled the end of the supply chain and the beginning of a defibrillator. After this moment—as the defibrillator was checked for trace helium, as it was sealed in two plastic trays and sterilized in a bath of ethylene oxide, as its box was stacked with others and shipped to hospitals across the world—it was a defibrillator. Even if ruined, it was a defective defibrillator. It was a thing. Before this, it was earth in the slow process of becoming.

If defibrillators are from a place the way a person is from a place—if the birth certificate is stamped and signed—then mine was from LA.

In his 1954 essay "The Question Concerning Technology," the German philosopher Martin Heidegger suggests that technology is not made, exactly, but revealed out of a set of conditions, letting "what is not yet present arrive into presencing." His concept of revealing recognizes, in the broadest way, all that must come together in the making of a thing. He points to four different "causes" of an object: the matter out of which it is made (*causa materialis*), the form or shape it becomes (*causa formalis*), the purpose that determines its form (*causa finalis*), and the actor who directly brings about the final form (*causa efficiens*). If a chalice is made of silver, writes Heidegger, silver is co-responsible for the chalice. The chalice is indebted, i.e., owes thanks to, the silver.

"But the sacrificial vessel is indebted not only to the silver," he continues, for it "appears in the aspect of a chalice and not that of a brooch or a ring. Thus the sacrificial vessel is at the same time indebted to the aspect (*eidos*) of chaliceness."

The vessel owes its existence, as well, to the need in the world for a thing that will perform the sacred function of the chalice, "within the realm of consecration and bestowal." And yet the chalice cannot become this combination of silver, the shape of the cup, and the aspect of sacredness without the *causa efficiens*: "The silversmith considers carefully and gathers together the three aforementioned ways of being responsible and indebted.... [They] owe thanks to the pondering of the silversmith."

In Heidegger's view, some things have the capacity to bring themselves forth—the way a flower blooms or a tree bears fruit, "the bursting open belonging to the bringing-forth." But a made object requires others to "cause" this bursting open.

It had been Heidegger's language that stunned me when first I read "The Question Concerning Technology." *The chalice owes thanks,* Heidegger said. *The chalice is indebted.* In the American life I led, objects were always showing up magically, complicit in questions of resource use that remained invisible even to those who held them. So much of what we touched we did not really *see,* much less with the reverence Heidegger offers.

Now I saw that the defibrillator, too, owed thanks: To mountains and smelters. To engineers and doctors and assembly workers. To the genetic mutation that demanded it and the body that accepted it. Here in the white-and-aqua hallways of St. Jude Medical, the defibrillator was revealed out of a set of conditions; here, the grand vision of using electricity to solve death met the practical constraints of putting a battery and capacitor and tiny computer inside a human body. Here, anonymous-looking metal and polymer parts came off the shipping dock and into the dream of saving lives.

Instead of silversmiths we had corporations: not responsible alone, but responsible.

Roy steered me down a long white hallway toward a line of manufacturing windows. In front of us a steady stream of people entered a doorway. "They're just getting off lunch," Roy said. He looked down at me. "Would you be okay going in? Meeting some of them?"

"Of course," I said.

"They don't get to meet patients often," he said. "It's pretty special for them."

At the entrance to the manufacturing floor, people were pulling long checkered gowns off a rack. Everyone had gauzy blue bonnets on their heads; some of the men wore beard nets. Roy called out to a younger man as he slipped in from the manufacturing floor. "Hey, Orem," he said. "You want to bring out those employees?"

A series of cubbyholes behind Roy's head held pairs of squishy-looking sandals. Clean shoes. "Are those Crocs?" I asked.

"Honey, this is California," Roy said. "They're Birkenstocks." And sure enough, I leaned forward to look, and the foam heels read BIRKI'S.

Originally, Roy told me as we waited, the Sylmar factory did everything except the defibrillator's microelectronics, which were assembled in Scottsdale. Then the insurance company—eyeing Sylmar's proximity to the San Fernando fault—said, "Uh, that's a $4 million revenue stream. Maybe you oughta think about spreading those eggs out." As of my visit, 50 percent of St. Jude defibrillators were made in Puerto Rico at the Arecibo plant, 40 percent were made in Sylmar, and 10 percent were made in Penang, Malaysia. "Those mostly service the Asian market," Roy said. "Mostly Chinese, Indian, the Middle East." Japan wouldn't buy from Malaysia because of old war wounds, so Sylmar filled the Japanese orders. He said the Liberty factory in South Carolina, which I'd also looked into visiting, was being expanded to handle pacemaker microelectronics.

Then, casually, Roy said, "Yours was made in Sylmar." This was as close as I would get to a serial-number trace, I thought, as he sang out the names of the factories—Sylmar, Scottsdale, Liberty—places that were, in their own way, inside my body. It felt strangely satisfying to know my device was not manufactured abroad. Roy told me the supervisor was gathering employees who actually worked on my defibrillator all those years ago, and we waited as the number of workers passing us thinned.

On a cool, sunny day nine months earlier, I'd driven from my home in Tucson to the Scottsdale facility Roy had named, a few hours north. If Sylmar was where my defibrillator was finally—at long last—born, the Scottsdale facility was where they'd made its unfinished brain. A squat, gray-tiled building with the same blue-green reflective entrance as Sylmar's, the Scottsdale facility was smaller. In a strangely intimate main room, the cubicles of administrative staff and engineers sat just feet from the long glass wall of the Clean Room, where employees in white hairnets moved ghostlike and soundless, epoxying microelectronics circuits. Every few hours, if the quality managers and engineers in cubicles looked up from their work, they might have seen the people in the Clean Room gather in a circle with their arms in the air, stretching left, then right, bending carefully at the waist, pinwheeling their hands.

In the Scottsdale Clean Room, everything was white or metal. The workers wore booties, beard nets, finger condoms, grounding straps. Air-conditioning flowed from vents on the ceiling year-round to make sure the temperature remained stable, and little sensors measured particulate matter. The environment needed to be controlled in every way—from humidity to pressurization—to keep any "killer defects" from getting into the circuits.

In the Clean Room they tortured the brains. Spun them, beat them, dropped them. The brains were put in hot centrifuges called burning boards. The brains were frozen. One, hit by a .45 slug, didn't explode. Another, exposed to an extreme temperature, reset.

Consider the limits of a human body. Consider it bending, pulling, riding bicycles, flying airplanes or jumping out of them. Consider it crumpled in car crashes, living on glaciers, getting in fistfights, traipsing over hot sand. Most humans who contained defibrillators did not do these things with regularity, yet some of us did, and it would be unforgivable if device failure occurred. To go in a human, the cyborg part must be *better* than human. The engineers must know at what point it fails. All defibrillators, already rock tortured into purity and shape, must pass tests of stamina.

There was the risk of the device firing when it should not. There was the risk of the device failing to go off when it must. There was the failure of epoxy, parts moving around, substances leaking into the body. There were brittle wires with coatings that, over time, cracked and rubbed.

The cost of one defibrillator contained all those that were discarded: a tax on ghost brains. Those that made the cut were sent on to Sylmar, for placement inside a titanium can.

All this is referred to as the Grandma Test. As in—*Would you put this in your grandma?*

The St. Jude–Sylmar employees formed a semicircle in front of me: Elsa, Maria, Ana, Cristina, Jeanette, Raoul. Roy introduced me, and we stood awkwardly smiling at each other. "Do you have any questions for her?" Roy said. Silence. "Okay, I know you're thinking it," Roy said finally, "so I'll ask: Has it gone off?"

"Only by accident," I said, swallowing. They didn't probe further, and it felt tinny to talk about it. "Last November," I offered. "I got shocked three times in a row." The employees nodded. I wished for their sake the answer was different, so I added, "My sister's once saved her life, though," and did not mention her accidental shocks. No one asked what it felt like, the typical next question, and so the silence hung.

"While everyone is here," Roy said, excited like a little kid, "we have something for you." He dug through his bottomless pockets, carefully sifting through sample ICDs and pacemakers, at last lifting one to his chest dramatically. "A special token of our gratitude," he said, and placed an ICD into my palm. I held it up to my chest instinctively, comparing the size, as he said, "This isn't the one you have now—

it's the one we hope you'll get next time," flashing a slightly absurd marketing grin. I turned the device over and saw the word *Ellipse* printed on one side, in the standard lettering I'd seen on each sample device he passed me. On the other side, my name was etched into the metal. *Katherine Standefer. September 23, 2013. Thank You From St. Jude Medical.*

It was surprisingly heavy—a sophisticated paperweight, cool when Roy took it from his pocket but quickly warming to my hand. I squeezed it in my palm to feel the curve of it.

"Do you have any questions for them?" Roy asked me, and my face flushed hot. *I wish I'd known ahead of time.* On the spot, I asked them their roles, and they went around the circle: issuing serial numbers, attaching the capacitor, X-ray and septum pictures, RF to hybrid, patching and fixing. Wet room. Laser welding. Listening to them, I realized I didn't even know what all these processes were.

"Elsa has been here the longest," someone said. Elsa shifted uncomfortably, a pale woman with a heavily lined but kind face, bright pink lipstick smudged across her lips.

"How long have you been here?" I asked.

"Since 1980," she said quietly. She had a thick accent.

"You've been doing this since before I was born!" I blurted, and she smiled uncomfortably again.

Another silence elapsed. Birki's shifted on the tiled floor.

"Do you all live nearby?" I said. "You don't have to commute across LA, do you?"

"No, I live right over there," Raoul said, "like real nearby." He gestured across his shoulder.

Jeanette smiled. "I drive from an hour away."

She lifted her hands. "I do it for you," she said, and everyone laughed.

"How did you hear about the job?" I asked. "Were you already familiar with St. Jude?" Everyone looked around at one another. Raoul stepped forward.

"For me, you know, I'd just gotten out of high school, and my friend, he said hey, St. Jude is hiring, so I thought, well, that sounds cool."

"Raoul is our manufacturing trainer," Roy said. "The goal for ICDs is to put out a new product every nine months. That usually has to do with a feature being approved by the FDA. Plus any new employees. He trains them, too."

"Does this job make you look at electronics differently?" I asked them. "Like cell phones? That you know what's inside?"

Mostly they shook their heads, shrugged, but Jeanette was nodding, her curly brown hair jostling beneath her hairnet. "Yeah, it does for me. I got that when I smashed my computer," she said, and laughed.

I almost asked to take a picture with them, but this seemed too much. All that really bridged us, awkwardly, was the device in my chest, which four years earlier their hands had carefully assembled, epoxied, tested. I thanked them, and so did Roy, and as they slipped away onto the manufacturing floor in their checkered smocks, I couldn't help but think how happy they all looked. They'd all been at St. Jude for years, and I couldn't stop thinking, *This was the old American Dream.* To graduate high school and get a good, steady manufacturing job. To work your way up, like Raoul. To play your part in saving lives.

The defibrillator owed them thanks. I felt weirdly happy, weirdly proud.

Around the bend we peered through the glass at a woman who sat inches from us, applying epoxy to the component parts, fitting them in. She pretended not to see us at first. Then her eyes flickered up to mine, and we both grinned, embarrassed, caught. Roy waved at her, and she waved back. He gestured behind her, to the woman looking at an ICD beneath an X-ray. "That's Raoul's wife," he said. "We love when people have interconnectedness here."

There were ninety-six steps to building an ICD on this manufacturing floor, Roy told me, pointing at a poster that grouped them into stages: Every part coming off the trucks went through inspection. A polymer coating called parylene coated the ICD "like dew" to one one-thousandth of an inch, protecting the electronic components from any moisture that might accidentally enter the titanium can. Before being laser-sealed, the half cans were tested at body temperature. "You put everything together and say, 'Give me 750 volts,'" Roy said. "If it gives you 770, you turn the settings down a bit to compensate for the natural 'offness' of the machine." Once the cans were welded shut (here, the bobble-gloves), they were tested for any remaining helium that could affect the ICD's electrical conductivity. The header—where the wire to the heart plugs into the device—was added. The device was tested again. Then the ICDs were cosmetically scratched, so that all would have the same uniform matte St. Jude look. They were examined under an X-ray. Finally, the ICDs were packaged in double trays, anticipating the moment in the operating room when the plastic would be peeled back on the container, when one nurse would hold the first plastic tray (its outside no longer sterile) and wait for a second nurse (already in a sterile operating environment) to pull the second tray out. Then the surgeon would lift and place the sealed can—a tortured metal brain that passed all the tests—inside a chest pocket. Inside a human being.

CHAPTER 4

Boulder, Colorado
2009

In those first days, I slept on the floor of my sister's Boulder sorority house on the Hill, rolling out my thin camping air mattress and blowing into its mouthpiece until it puffed. The hallways were full of girls with glossy, highlighted hair, their mascara flawless, their sandals matching their shirts.

I found myself examining my eyebrows far more than usual. I slept the three allowed nights at the foot of her desk.

During the day I filled out job applications and perused housing listings at the Boulder Public Library, one hourlong slot at a time. My computer—ancient and nicknamed Apple-eptic—was in the shop. Sometimes, while Christine was at her restaurant job scooping noodles into bowls and ringing people up, I borrowed her laptop, working from the coffee shop beside Alpha Chi. But she seemed resistant, wary of me. She needed her laptop. She lived a busy life. What I needed was more than what she had to offer.

I joined instead the small group of people who haunted the library computer queue: the other unemployeds, the elderly, the middle schoolers who burst inside in jostling packs. Out front, people experiencing homelessness clustered on the lawn, their bags rumpled and their eyes yellowed, muttering as they slipped by me to the bathroom. For the first time I could see the way a life came unwound. The way illness could mean one month without a job, then another—the way bills could take you under. How once things started to happen to you, it got harder to get up.

But for the grace of my father, I thought. My own accounts would soon be empty. What kept me from chaos was a matter only of whom I had been born to, and how they were willing to keep me.

At the library I applied for every professional job I saw and every service job with insurance. I made seven different versions of my résumé and walked up and down Pearl Street placing them into the hands of people at bookstores and bars. Beneath my cheerful smile, there was a dangerous buzzing in me. The unraveling that comes with constant fear.

At the river a man peeled away from the circle of his group, took a half step toward me, and jeered, "And how are *you,* little lady," angling his head to catch my eyes. It was as though he could see inside me. How I tipped at some edge.

In those weeks I learned that "garden apartment" was code for *disappointing basement.* I filed into these dark and damp rooms, tailing property managers, looking for the place that would provide me an address for my driver's license, key to establishing residency. Looking for the place I would recover, close enough to walk for groceries in the weeks after surgery when driving wouldn't be allowed. Looking for a place that could order my life.

You can complain if the undergrads upstairs are loud, one property manager shrugged. You can call the police.

The good news, another said, was that Boulder had made it illegal to pull couches out onto the grass. I looked again at the bathroom floor. I wasn't sure whether or not it was rotting.

My mother flew in under the assumption that I would have an apartment to move into. I did not. Together, we visited disappointing basements. We slept in the ground-floor guest room of the sorority house, and all night the drunk students smoked on the ledge outside, their conversations coming in our open window, the night punctuated by giggles and shouts. In the morning, bleary and hot, we drove the neighborhoods within walking distance of downtown looking for FOR RENT signs that weren't on Craigslist. We sought the inexpensive, but never forgot that I would be recovering from heart surgery—that in one of these rooms I would spend long hours in pain.

The house on Maxwell Avenue was a Victorian split into four apartments, gray-green with a deep red door. There was a giant maple out front, the kind of tree I instantly wanted to wrap my arms around, to lean into, pressing my forehead against its bark. Under my hand it pulsed with a kind of intelligence.

When Mom and I arrived early for the showing, a Siamese cat wound across the single cement step. We circled the house, peering into its windows: beautiful wood floors and historic molding. A shared backyard with a table and chairs, room for a composter, maybe a tiny garden. I could feel myself lean in: I was planning.

The property manager arrived frantic, apologizing. She took us up the stairs and let us into number 4.

Right away I knew. "It's perfect," I breathed. The windows, long and thin, stretched almost from ceiling to floor in the middle of each wall. On such a September day, the maple leaves clustered toward the window, and the green light made me feel like I was in a treehouse.

"This is it," I said, running my hands over the old gas stove.

When I turned to the property manager to ask when I could move in—ready to haul bags up from the car that instant—she raised her eyebrows at me. "First your background check will have to clear," she said. "Then you'll need to come in and sign the lease. Are you employed?"

"No," I said. "I just moved to town." She sighed. I would need a cosigner.

"So there's no way she could move in this weekend?" my mother asked.

No, the manager said, looking impatient, explaining to us that she was trying to leave town for Labor Day. "And anyway it'll take a business day to get the background check back, and then you'll have to fax in the cosigner's form, and *then* you'll have to come in to sign the lease and get the key." No one would be in the office over the holiday weekend, she said.

Mom and I looked at each other. "So much for coming to town to help you move," she said.

As we drove away, we consoled ourselves: the grocery store was a half-mile walk down the hill. The hospital sat beside it. And Maxwell Avenue climbed steeply west toward Mount Sanitas, dead-ending exactly half a mile away—in the parking lot of Dr. Oza's practice.

The wait would be worth it.

All weekend, as my mother and I bought dishes at a thrift store and looked for a bed, a hot rage flickered through me. The packed stop-lights. The ringing of jackhammers. The stupid undergrads, clouds of them, zipping dangerously in front of cars on their longboards. Boulder was a busy, hot hell. I wanted to go home. I found myself snapping at my mom, at one point getting out of the car at a stoplight so she could drive, too overwhelmed by decisions.

"I feel like I'm being punished!" she cried out.

On the radio, politicians calmly explained why extending health care to millions would ruin the country. They spoke of nonexistent "death panels" that would decide whether or not people received lifesaving care, without understanding that they were, at that very minute, acting as *my* death panel.

"No one in America should go broke because they get sick," President Barack Obama wrote in a *New York Times* editorial eighteen days before I moved to Boulder to access heart surgery. That year 60 percent of bankruptcies would be attributable to medi-cal bills—most of those toppled were well-educated, middle-class homeowners—and nearly forty-five thousand Americans would die from being uninsured.

I sat in the passenger seat with my face in my hands. I did not want the life I had been handed.

At the end of the weekend, I dropped my exhausted mother at the air-port and checked into the University Inn, a sallow green motel with a thin white metal rail running along each floor. The hotel sat at the bottom of the Hill, where campus transitioned into downtown, just a few blocks from the library.

The first time I turned into the parking lot, a woman stood scream-ing in a window on the first floor, her curtains drawn wide open, hands dangling at her hips. She had the tough skin of a smoker, hollowed cheeks. I watched her mouth move violently, soundlessly, from inside my car. Her shoulders shook, tired-looking bleached hair piled on her head. Was she talking to someone I couldn't see?

I put the car in Park and craned my head around, trying to see. No one.

The parking lot was mostly empty, and when I got out I could hear her muffled voice against the glass. I tried not to look again, not to stare, stepping quickly toward reception, but her muffled, crackling voice followed me, would not shake loose.

The next morning, as I went to retrieve free breakfast from the buffet against the office wall, a big man stood solidly next to her door, talking quietly. He had a buzz cut and fat black sideburns. At his feet, the remnants of the night: a plate of little square hamburgers, cigarette butts, aluminum foil folded into a plastic Lunchables tray. The woman hunched as she brought more trash out. She was quiet, but more broken-looking.

Her face would come to me over and over. The violent shape of a screaming mouth, muffled by glass. Wondering what was she on. What was she doing in that motel.

In the morning I checked out of the motel and buried myself back in the over-air-conditioned library. *Public and Tribal Lands Stewardship Intern. Spa Attendant. Barista. Undergraduate Admissions Counselor. Dispatcher for Safe Walk Program. Substitute Preschool Teacher. Server.* The résumés went out. I prayed someone would read them. It was hard to believe that I had only been in town one week; these Boulder days seemed tumorous. I ducked out of the library to take calls from Sam, who had started calling me three times a day. Otherwise we felt disconnected, and squabbled.

"Are you sure you don't want me to come?" he had asked the morning I loaded my car.

I'd shaken my head. "No use having two of us in limbo," I said. "I don't know what's going to happen. You need to work. You can come once there's an apartment." I still thought it was true. But now I felt the gap opening between us. Five hundred miles northwest, he still woke in our bed beneath Snow King Mountain, the valley cool and socked in with rain. He drank coffee out of our mugs in our dark wooden boat of a living room. He diced vegetables from our farm share. In some way, my life went on without me there, and I imagined myself, like a ghost, setting water over the burner to boil, or heading off into the pine woods with a group of hikers. Maybe I should just get in the car and drive the eight hours home, I thought, picturing our gravel drive, my hands in Sam's sun-bleached hair. But what would it solve? I was still far from being a Colorado resident, still nowhere near surgery.

The first business day passed without a call from the property manager. I returned to the University Inn, to a different tired room. Here the days began to string together. My parents worried that if they guaranteed the lease for me, it would somehow come to light when the hospital evaluated my need for financial aid, and would disqualify me. My best friend from college, Makendra, the only twenty-five-year-old I knew who was a homeowner, offered to cosign. But she worked for a wild horse advocacy organization, and that summer there were roundups on the Forest Service land in the Pryor Mountains of north-central Wyoming, so she sent her faxes at night to the property management company from a motel in Lovell, on the edge of the wilderness—faxes that arrived only in parts, first all signature and no agreement, then all agreement and no signature. Then one of the faxes finally went through—her work was done—but a top manager was required to sign all leases. He wasn't in. And wasn't in. And then he was, but there was no key. Each morning I put my things into my car. Each day I called the property manager from the library, and each night I returned after the close of business hours to the University Inn, poured wine into plastic cups. The apartment shifted into a mirage. The surgery receded into impossibility.

One evening, a crowd of drunk boys passed loudly through the parking lot of the University Inn. I went to the window. In the entire motel, only three of us were looking. Me. The clerk, stepping out of the office with his hands on his hips. And the screaming woman. She pointed and hollered at them, swaying on the sidewalk outside her room. Then she turned, sighted me on the second floor, and shrieked. Jabbing her finger over and over at me. Her mouth violently open.

I backed quickly away from the blinds.

The next afternoon I went to my one-month checkup with Dr. Oza. Despite all the problems I'd had with beta-blockers, in light of my sister's lifesaving shock he raised my dosage again.

After the appointment, flattened, I called Sam, crying. I did not want that hard fist of metal inside me, or a lifetime hitched to the American medical system, which I was now excluded from as a matter of policy. But having it implanted was my only hope for going off those stranglingly high doses of beta-blockers. Having it implanted seemed my only chance of feeling safe again. Once inside me, the ICD would be watching my heart all the time, a computer that counted beats per minute and recorded high heart rates, theoretically distinguishing between dangerous and normal rhythms. But even if I didn't receive shocks, every three months I would need to have the system checked, the computer's recordings downloaded. I would never again be just a flesh being. In the back of the cardiology office, they would hook me to a computer to check my settings. They would use its buttons to race and palpitate my heart, making sure the device could still control it, looking for the sudden changes in resistance or responsiveness that meant something had happened to my device or wires. I would never again walk through an airport metal detector. I would never have an MRI.

I didn't want it.

But I did not understand how I was supposed to live with death staring me down like that, if I went without it. How I would live with these climbing doses of a drug that left me limp and out of breath. How I was supposed to do normal things, and not always expect to die.

It was too much. I needed a reminder, I told him, of why my life was worth saving.

* * *

My room that night backed up to the strip of park along Boulder Creek, and the sound of the men in the park along the creek came in through the window more loudly than before. I could hear the men shaking out old comforters. Men who were once children, I knew. Men who were once boys. Who sat in classrooms. Who played. What the world had done to them. How the world had failed them.

The laughter that came through my window did not feel safe. Did not feel like laughter.

I leaned against the headboard, holding a mug of wine. I had been crying for hours. I had been on the phone with my mother telling her I did not want to live.

"What are you going to do?" she asked me, fear in her voice, and I couldn't answer. But I stared at the bottle of heart medication on the orange bedspread beside me, and I knew I could take them all. Beta-blockers. A drug that had, as its side effect, low blood pressure. Vasodilation. I could go limp in this world. I could block out the men whose lives had shrunk to the banks of the river, the crazy woman with her frizzled hair and wild late-night grief. I could block out the life I had loved, gone now.

I saw it clearly: what could fix the threat of my own death was death.

Five hundred miles northwest of me, Sam was arriving at board game night.

Then my phone rang. It was a student from the private liberal arts college I'd gone to, just calling to update my address. I began to cry. Then to laugh. "I don't know," I told her. "I have no fucking clue what my address is."

"Are you in a position to contribute to the annual fund?" she asked sweetly, politely.

"No," I said. "No, I'm waiting to have heart surgery, and I can't find a job." I wept into my hands, the phone cradled against my shoulder. Full of the distance between the self I was in that hotel room and the self I had been in college. "That college is the nicest place you'll ever be," I told her. "Good luck to you."

I hung up and lay on the bed, extinguished. The bottle of pills on the bed beside me.

And then a voice inside me said, *Put on your shoes.*

The voice said, *Go to the bookstore. Right now.*

I walked down Broadway. Stepped onto the Pearl Street Mall, with its humming bars and teens eating ice cream and men playing guitar for tips, and into the glittering storefront of the Boulder Book Store. I bought a copy of *The Amazing Adventures of Kavalier & Clay* and another of *The Alchemist.* I read them.

In this way, I lived until morning.

The next day, with forty minutes left until the end of business hours, the call would come. I would race from the library back to my car, tears leaking, speeding out east to 55th Street, floating up the steps of the property management company. I would sign the form. I would cup the cool keys in my palm. I would drive to Maxwell Avenue, sling a backpack over my shoulder, and let myself slowly into the apartment, looking at the long windows and sweet wooden floors with a sort of awe. Calling the futon guys for delivery. Calling Sam to say, Finally. Laying myself down on the floor just to say Mine.

With the key would come an electricity bill. With the key would come an account at the credit union down the street. The next week, clenching new statements bearing my address in my hand, I would drive to the DMV to become a resident.

And a month and a half later, when I arrived at the emergency room late one night with chest pains, I would hand them a Colorado driver's license.

Sam arrived the next evening from Jackson to stay for a few weeks, his car packed with my kitchen table, my big comfy chair, my little nightstand, my printer, all the furniture I had dragged across the country with me for years like quiet family members. I had not, until that moment, realized what it meant to own belongings with that kind of history. To get to keep them with you, the objects that tell your stories.

I ran out to meet him in the street. Back upstairs, he held two hands behind his back. "Pick a hand," he said, and I poked his right elbow. He drew forward a small black box, and my heart stopped. But inside was a small velvet bag, with delicate lavender earrings, which he slid into the holes of my ears, as I laughed.

"Taking your chances, eh?" I teased him. He once told me his girlfriends always broke up with him after he bought them jewelry. At Thanksgiving the previous year, we'd gone shopping in downtown Chicago at the Christkindlmarket with my parents, and he'd stared longingly at the pair of earrings I was trying on. "I wish I could buy you those," he said, "but I won't." He paid for our chocolate-covered strawberries, at equal cost.

Now we looked at each other in the empty apartment in Boulder as I slid them out of my ears to look at them: metal wheels lined with dark lavender beads. "They're beautiful," I said, putting them back in.

He smiled and told me a friend of ours had made them. "She said she'll do free maintenance if you break them," he teased me.

"You know me, don't you?"

He kissed me for a long time, our bags on the ground around us. Then he fell to his knees and gently put his face beneath my skirt.

In late September, after nearly a month of ceaseless job applications, I finally got a call back for a position I was excited about: investigative assistant at a criminal defense law firm that specialized in death row appeals. The lawyer who interviewed me was tall, young, and attractive, with a perfectly arranged head of brown hair. We met in a small, dark room in a business park on the east side of town, where he told me his client had been convicted of murder and sentenced to death in a fairly well-known case several years earlier. The job mostly involved watching long hours of security camera footage and reinterviewing witnesses, he said, possibly traveling to prisons or the neighborhood where the crime was committed. We'd be combing the case evidence for new details or irregularities. And if we found anything substantial, I might need to testify in court.

The work sounded painstaking. But as someone who obsessively followed questions, who loved to interview and write and speak publicly, I was thrilled. It was a job that would feel like more than just a way to become a resident.

Later that day I received an e-mail inviting me to write a letter about why I'd be well suited for the position. That night, I stood alone in the still-bare apartment and spoke aloud: "I want this job." I said it loudly, with intention, with no room for argument.

I got the job.

After a few weeks in Boulder, Sam returned to our cabin in Wyoming. Having him in town those first weeks in the apartment had been surprisingly hard. There were ways in which we were going through this together—and there were ways in which I lived this story alone. For Sam, the silver lining of my move to Boulder had been proximity to the Flatirons: long, iconic sandstone faces that overlooked town. With lots of old college friends and outdoor-industry contacts located in Boulder, Sam went out climbing with a friend all day on several occasions while he was in town. Then at night, when I asked him to go for a walk with me, he'd say no—he was too wiped out.

I'd burst into tears: wiped out! I would give anything to be wiped out from something vigorous—from fresh air and sweat—rather than woozy from beta-blockers.

When Sam invited me along with his cousin or buddies, I'd say yes just to be with him, driving north along the foothills to some clutch of boulders in an aspen grove. But then when I sat nearby journaling or reading, he'd get sad that I wasn't climbing. It was hard to explain to him the terror that had entered my life. Sudden spikes of adrenaline were the greatest risk for type 2 long QT syndrome, and though physical exertion wasn't itself a threat, climbing for me had always involved those moments when a toe suddenly slipped, I gasped, my heart ratcheted up, and sweat burst from my palms. Before, I'd known how to calm myself in these moments. Now, I understood I could pass out on the rock—if not from cardiac arrest, then from the beta-blockers limiting how well my heart could respond to the sudden exertion. What Sam loved best had become something that panicked me, and a loss between us.

Most of the time, though, we inhabited a sweet little world all our own. In Boulder we spent afternoons working at the BookEnd, a little café attached to the Boulder Book Store. The magazine Sam had worked for—the one that folded in the recession—had been purchased by another publisher; now he was collaborating part-time with the new editors to get it up and running, and freelancing on the side.

We were on a mission to find the best Indian restaurants in town. He brought me banana bread at the library when I got hungry. At night, we blared a sex-and-love-advice podcast while we cooked.

"Cheer up! I can think of a million things that aren't climbing that I want to do with you," he wrote in an e-mail from Jackson. But I felt an uneasiness at his reassurances, for in other moments he'd make some remark about how he couldn't imagine traveling internationally for any reason other than climbing, and I would see the alternative future I was trying to build for us—one that worked around my heart condition—become tepid and hazy again.

During Sam's September visit to Boulder, we'd gotten a call from our Jackson landlord. She told us she'd received a request for a housing reference from my apartment application and wanted to know what was going on. Rather than being put out, she confessed she was hoping to move back into her own house for the winter. She offered to let us move out just for six months. If we wanted, we could come back in June. We'd have first dibs.

The prospect of loosening our connection to Jackson was scary. But Sam was pleased by how many friends he had in Boulder, and we knew long distance would be hard around the procedure.

We decided: he would come to Colorado in late October with another load of our belongings, and we would return to Jackson together after that—to pack up the rest of the house and bring our lives south by trailer.

It was the end of the beginning for us, the start of something I did not know.

Up in Wyoming, Beating Heart Bear's light burned out. Sam found a tiny compass at the local gear store with a light that glowed red when you pressed it.

By text, he sent pictures, his surgery reports:

Beating Heart Bear's left leg seam, opened from the back.

Burned-out bulb pulled out.

New compass light inserted.

The bear carefully stitched shut.

The chest glowing red.

In Boulder, I laughed, then cried in relief. Not just that the bear's surgery had worked, which seemed to bode well for mine, but that the man had bought a light for the bear, opened him so carefully, had stitched so steadily. Had so tenderly held a small body in need, with his hands.

The job was a weight lifted; I'd earned the right to do something other than write cover letters. I'd also run into an old writing friend from college on the Pearl Street Mall, and now we met in coffee shops to give each other prompts.

Still, some nights the grief of what I'd lost, my fears about the procedure, took over, and I'd call Sam crying, drinking hot whiskey in bed. Sometimes I hung up on him, turned the phone off, and thought about ending my life again, and when I called him back, his voice was subdued.

"Hi."

"Lady's crazy," I said.

"I know." And there was nothing singsongy to it anymore. He wasn't going to talk me out of the assessment; we were tired of this.

We tried to make the distance funny, licking our phones, talking about the sex we would have when he arrived. After we hung up, I'd make myself get dressed and walk downtown to watch live music and write. Around other people, I didn't want to kill myself quite so much.

One drizzly morning, after a work meeting canceled, I texted my sister. Did she want to meet me at a piercing shop on the Hill, down the block from the sorority house? She did. She'd been thinking about getting a forward helix piercing—the cartilage rim at the front of her ear.

For weeks I had been drawing a dot on my nose and rushing periodically back into the bathroom to look at myself, angling my head. I had never been pulled toward body modifications before; I was thus far untattooed, my only piercing a conventional set of ear holes. But something felt different now. Urgent. To make a mark upon my body that I wanted. In late morning, Christine and I filled out our forms, looking nervously at studs. Then, in a small room in back, an attendant made Sharpie dots on my nose. Christine squeezed my hand as the attendant pushed the needle in.

I felt a rush of nausea. My eyes filled with tears. But Christine and I both knew there was worse to come for me.

The morning I got the e-mail from my new boss at the law firm, Sam was back in town. We'd just finished making love, our faces red and skin warmed, and I was about to be late for a writing date.

Although I don't like making this decision, the lawyer wrote, *I don't believe that we are a good match and have found through experience that it is better to separate early when those indicators are present...*

"No. No no no no no."

"What is it?" Sam rushed into the room. I turned the computer toward him and pointed, my head spinning, my breath coming in gasps. "Oh, my god," he said. "Do you think there's anything you can do?" I shook my head. That was it.

I hadn't even received a paycheck. I was back on the same cliff.

As Sam folded me into his chest, he began to cry, too. ("It was the most upset I've ever seen you," he told me later.)

I was going to die before I got the surgery, I thought. I was never going to get my life back.

When I left to go write with Liza, Sam kept saying, "Be good. Be good." As though I would not be coming back.

I called Dr. Oza's nurse from the coffee shop, standing outside in the October chill. I had gotten a job and lost it. I was a voter and a driver. This had to count as residency. It had to.

"I just want to schedule it," I told the nurse. "I can't do this anymore. What are the next dates?"

"Are you sure?" she said. "I just want you to be careful. A patient with health insurance got his surgery the other day, and even though the company paid 90 percent, he wound up with a bill for $18,000."

"Emily, this just has to end," I said. I asked her about the Colorado Indigent Care Program, the one she and Dr. Oza had mentioned before I moved—whether it was something I could count on.

"I wish I could guarantee they'd accept you," she said. "But you have to submit the bill afterward. There's no preapproval."

"I'll just declare bankruptcy." I wept into my hand. "There's nothing to take but my car." Emily was quiet for a moment.

"I'm not telling you this," she said. "I mean, I can't recommend this. We never had a conversation about this. But if you were to come in through the emergency room, you'd be the most likely to get aid."

"Really?"

"Yes," she said. "That is where the hospital writes off the most bills. It's just how the system works. I mean, say you had another syncope. Say you came in having passed out. Maybe you forgot to take your beta-blocker. There would really be no way for them to know…I never told you this." She paused. "Dr. Oza's out of town right now." It was a Thursday, and he did procedures on Mondays and Tuesdays. "This week won't work anyway. Think about it."

"My parents are coming into town tomorrow for Christine's birthday and parents' weekend," I said. "We'll talk about it. But maybe October twenty-seventh?"

"That is possible," she said. "But be careful."

I have been advised to fake cardiac arrest, I thought. It was ridiculous. It was brilliant. It would be as simple as not taking my beta-blocker. It would be as simple as going for a run.

And I was on the grassy slopes already in my mind, sprinting uphill as though my life depended on it. Running, gasping. Praying for collapse.

A few days later, on the morning after Christine's twenty-first birthday, my parents and I took a long walk down the Boulder Creek path, waiting for her to wake up. "So how would this work?" my mom said. "I book a flight in advance but pretend I booked it last-minute? I just don't tell anyone?"

The creek burbled peacefully. Yellow leaves dropped slowly around us.

"I just think it sounds too dangerous, Kati," my dad said.

"I'm not sure I'm comfortable lying," my mom said. "Sam would have to lie, too."

"I don't know," I said. "I just don't know what to do. It's been too long."

"We'll keep thinking about it," Mom said. "October twenty-seventh?"

"October twenty-seventh. Maybe."

But the panic passed; my financial fears loomed larger than my impatience. I did not call in to book a surgery, and Sam did book a U-Haul, and near the end of October we drove north to Jackson, packed up our sweet boat-cabin, met our friends at the brewery to say goodbye, and headed out. We woke at 3:00 a.m. in the frost, loading the last of the furniture with cold knuckles. Rolled through the silent town, blue with night. I'd grieved two months before, but this was different, more final. And yet Sam was with me this time, gripping the steering wheel against the gusts of morning wind, smiling at me from time to time. The rivers were steaming in the dawn, the last aspens yellow in the curves of those high mountains.

The trailer could go only fifty-five miles per hour, and the drive took so long that by the time we arrived we had only a few hours to get the trailer back. Sam called his cousin, who was an undergraduate at the university, and the two of them flew up and down the stairs with boxes, bookcases, skis. We knew some of it would have to go right to the storage unit my mom and I had opened.

I carried what I could but kept finding myself spinning, beta-blocked, almost dropping things. I knocked my hand between the furniture and the doorjamb, swearing. Finally I settled into making room for their next dump, restacking boxes, beginning to worry about the amount of stuff we were trying to fit in this tiny apartment.

Finally, at 11:00 p.m., we lay down in bed, exhausted. Sam's body settling in beside me. With the lights off, Jackson seemed already a distant memory.

Then the chest pains started.

I said nothing at first. Bodies are weird, I told myself. It's nothing.

But then it became like god herself was sitting on my chest. A heavy, dark sensation.

"Sam," I said finally. "I'm having really bad chest pain."

He lay silently beside me for a moment before speaking. "What do you want to do?"

"I'm sure I'll be fine," I said. "I just thought I should tell you." In case, I thought. We lay in the darkness.

"Do you need water?" he asked.

"I don't think so," I said.

If anyone walked into the room then, they might have thought we were sleeping. Both of us with our eyes shut, leaning into each other. The sounds of breath.

I wanted it to be nothing. I wanted to fall asleep. I wanted to stop being such a drag on Sam's life. I wanted the drama to end. But I had to be honest. "I'm really scared," I said.

"Get dressed," he said. "That's it. We're going to the hospital." I wanted to argue, to assuage him. But I knew. We turned the light back on. We dressed between rows of boxes. This time I took my stuffed bears with me, not knowing when we would come home.

My parents, lying in bed in the Midwest, picked up the phone call from Sam. It was after midnight. The date was October 26.

When my father hung up, he turned to my mother. "Either she's lying," he said, "or this is an act of god."

The hospital kept me overnight. In the morning, Dr. Oza came in and sat quietly before my bed. "Were you able to make your arrangements?" he said.

I found myself chattering. *Maybe, maybe,* I found myself saying. Telling him about the artist in Jackson I'd modeled for dozens of times over the years, who'd offered to fund-raise for me when I saw her briefly the week before. "There's so much money in this valley," she said, suggesting they could auction off paintings of me that people had done over the years.

The artist's idea was the kind of lovely offer that bubbled up and then disappeared; it was nothing to make medical decisions on. Within weeks, the artist would have her own family crisis to attend to. In the meantime, I had no job, no insurance, no real guarantees. The only arrangement I'd made was becoming a Colorado resident.

Dr. Oza listened calmly. When I finished, he smiled slightly. "What would you like me to do?" he asked.

In a sense, the decision had been made long ago, when I quit my life in Jackson. Yet even at this point, it felt like a decision, a choice after which my body would never be the same. I did not want a computer in me. I felt this with a spiritual certainty I could not explain. And I feared that after I got it, I wouldn't have access to the health-care systems that were supposed to take care of it. Nothing had changed in all this.

Yet I was also hungry for it. I was tired of being afraid, tired of putting my life on hold. The life I loved had fallen apart. Here, finally, was a way back to the world of the living.

I looked at Dr. Oza and was so afraid.

"Put it in," I said.

CAUSA MATERIALIS

CHAPTER 5

Moramanga, Madagascar
2014

O utside the boomtown of Moramanga, the hills pushed up like long, grassy shoulder blades. It was winter in the Southern Hemisphere, winter in the highlands of Madagascar. In the flat places at the base of the hills, rice paddies gleamed green. Above them, old men, barefoot, urged zebu up steep ridges. Women carried mahampy baskets on their heads. My guide, Anja, and I had met at the mining company's interpretive center in town, and now we drove up the long red road toward the nickel and cobalt pit in a jostling company truck. The clouds hung low and dark, light bursting between their cracks, a kind of chest-aching beautiful.

The mine was young. On the day I visited, it had been in production for only five months, although seven years had elapsed since construction began. Mineral exploration at the deposit dated back to 1960. Companies kept handing the project off to one another, until finally in 2006 the government finalized its environmental impact assessment and issued permits to Ambatovy—a joint venture between South Korean, Japanese, and Canadian mining companies and the largest-ever foreign investment on the island. Expected to produce 60,000 tonnes of refined nickel, 5,600 tonnes of cobalt, and 210,000 tonnes of ammonium sulfate (a fertilizer), the mine required the removal of a village and the dismantling of a forest ecosystem home to endangered species found nowhere else in the world.

I had cobalt in my battery, nickel in my microelectronics.

If it wasn't yet, this was about to be the largest lateritic nickel mine in the world. Lateritic, meaning: weathered rock. Meaning limestone, sandstone, or clay, leaching over time into the ground as water percolated, leaving behind what was less soluble: nickel, cobalt, iron, copper. The ore was soft, permeable. Two separate deposits draped across 1,600 hectares—nearly three thousand football fields—each twenty to one hundred meters deep. Bulldozers removed overburden with their swooped noses. Articulated haul trucks shuttled the red dirt to the Ore Preparation Plant. For every one thousand kilograms of red earth at this mine, there lay ten kilograms of nickel and a single kilogram of cobalt.

When it rained, the soft earth ran downhill off the road and clogged the rice paddies. The company knew a certain amount of this was inevitable. They paid the farmers when it happened. It was in the budget. To make a road cut was to release the earth: to make a wound that would not reliably stop leaking.

Some of the farmers were relocated because of the road, because of their ruined rice paddies. For others, the company held zebu sacrifices, where they drank rum together. It was in the budget. When I heard these stories, I wondered whom they sent, on behalf of the corporation, to bring the zebu. To drink the rum. To watch the gullet split.

The road climbed. Now greenery, tangled and tall, began to mount on the roadsides. Suddenly we had left the long silver hills for a dense wet world. Lemur bridges arced over the road. The canopy cut the light. Everything was splattered with red mud. The trucks, passing through all day, sent up titan clouds of dust, truck after truck after truck.

Company biologists counted the lemurs, Anja told me. They knew how many crossed the bridges. Sifakas, with their black faces and white fluffy heads; indris, with their tufted ears and fierce eyes and little opposable thumbs, some tagged with radio collars. The biologists tracked how many crossed the bridges and charted which tree hollows the lemurs used. They held the soft primates in their arms to bloodlet them, so they could monitor their health.

When the forest came down, they left it half chopped to give the animals time to leave. A compassionate pause. The machines cut, wait, cut, wait. Their engines a roar of warning. When the bulldozers finally came, the biologists "manually salvaged" any lemurs who had not left. To "manually salvage" was to knock at the tree like a houseguest, to scoop lemurs from the wreckage. They hoped the lemurs would use the bridges. They hoped the lemurs would use the protected forest corridor, which would deliver them to Andasibe-Mantadia National Park or the forest known as Ankerana, where they could find a new home.

In the company's plan there would be "no net loss."

A truck drove by spraying water. Dust control, Anja said. One cannot open the red heart of a mountain and expect it will not bleed.

It had taken me six months to find the mine I wanted to visit and another ten to raise the funds to go. Near my home in Arizona, I had peered over the edge at closed copper pits, marbled purple and pink, now fenced-off tourist attractions. I'd visited the old smelter up the highway—sentineled by eroding walls of tailings—which used to finish copper anodes and send them by train to a refinery in Amarillo. On a road trip through Wyoming the summer after my shocks, I'd driven through the Rattlesnake Hills looking for a new gold mine reportedly in development, only to discover the whole center of the state a reclamation pit from when uranium boomed in the '70s. The reconstructed hills, chalky yellow-white, had been graded into shelves, with grass and erosion grooves in neat rows. What had grown there looked fake; makeup over a scar that had never healed. The earth was as pockmarked as the moon with our digging.

I didn't find the gold mine, but I did find the Rattlesnake Hills themselves: rimmed with stacks of rock like perfect disks, stumpy piñon pines, the orange stain of lichen. I left my car on the road and scrambled up. I ducked into a cave, the air sweet and cool despite the hot sun, and smelling sweetly of sage. I prayed the gold would not be, as the industry termed it, "economically recoverable."

By then, my research confirmed it: even if we ignored conflict minerals, there was a lot of bad news in mining. In Papua New

Guinea, security guards at a Barrick Gold Corporation mine gang-raped more than 130 local women. In South Africa, thirty-four miners striking at the Marikana platinum mine in protest of low wages (despite soaring profits) were shot by police in minutes. At the Grasberg copper mine in Indonesia, residents of Pasir Hitam abandoned their village because it was being eclipsed by mine waste. The Batu Hijau copper and gold mine, on the Indonesian island of Sumbawa, dumps forty million tons of mine waste containing heavy metals into the Senunu Bay of the Indian Ocean each year. And all over the world, women and children comb the slag piles outside the gates of industrial gold mines, hauling crushed ore into their homes, rolling mercury through the silt to separate out the gold, then heating the amalgam to disappear the mercury, leaving a tiny, pure gold bar. Day after day their homes fill with a mercurial vapor that causes tremors, body numbness, vomiting, irritability, lowered intelligence, even paralysis—damaging entire communities.

The stories came from all corners of the world and in every variety imaginable. I understood it would be impossible to learn what stories this precise ICD—the one in my body—carried. And even if I could, by the time I learned, I'd be on to the next device, subject to the buzz of low battery. It felt like the opposite of an acquittal: instead, each defibrillator, repository of so many minerals from around the world, could be implicated in so much. I wondered if I should view mining's bad news as inevitable, chalk it up to the involvement of human beings. After all, there isn't a corner of the planet where we're immune from corruption, depravity, desperation. Yet it seemed more complicated than that, as though extraction is uniquely connected to human pain. Perhaps because it's such hard work that exploiting human beings seems like a reasonable option: to ease your own load if you are a warlord, to keep costs down if you are a capitalist. Perhaps because of the way extraction tends to concentrate men in isolated camps where pressure builds, where drugs make long or painful shifts possible, where boredom begs to be eased. Perhaps because a lucrative mine gives repressive governments the cash cow they need to stay in power. Perhaps it's the way mining dangles a promise in vulnerable places—the way it leaves its scraps out for the most desperate to scramble over.

Was a defibrillator, lifesaving though it could be, a deal with a particular kind of devil? I found myself, in the year and a half of research between taking those shocks and landing in Madagascar, wondering whether a different story existed, whether through a hundred policies and procedures mining might be made more just.

That's how I found Ambatovy, one oppressively hot afternoon in Tucson, looking up mineral after mineral online trying to understand what it took to pull metal from the ground. Ambatovy seemed to be the rare mining project celebrated for its corporate social responsibility program, despite being located in one of the world's most cash-poor and biodiversity-rich countries. By the time I stumbled across the company's 2012 sustainability report, I'd read more than my fair share of the sleek brochures corporations produce to showcase their conscience and compliance. Too often, the documents featured celebratory pictures of sweaty people at a Fun Run, the corporate logo stamped on their T-shirts, raising money for a cause unrelated to the business. Or they focused on a new recycling initiative in the headquarters cafeteria—an action that looked good on paper but was peripheral to the real material impacts of the business.

At my table in a dim Tucson coffee shop, I read in Ambatovy's report about the Global Reporting Initiative, an international standards nonprofit that has built a framework of inquiry to help organizations voluntarily identify the "risks and opportunities" of their projects. Businesses like Ambatovy track down the answers to specific questions about their environmental, social, human rights, and governance repercussions under the philosophy that "you can't manage what you don't measure." Instead of making money and then giving some away, GRI's concept of "materiality" demands that companies ask themselves how they make their money and use their resources to address impacts at that point.

Ambatovy was also a pilot project for the Business and Biodiversity Offsets Programme (BBOP)—initiated by an NGO called Forest Trends—which required following a "mitigation hierarchy" to manage the mark of carving into endemic jungle. The mitigation hierarchy mandated that they first avoid ecosystem impacts whenever possible; then minimize whatever was unavoidable; then restore whatever had been affected; then finally offset what couldn't be restored. So, too, was Ambatovy obligated to follow the Equator Principles, a credit risk management framework required by ninety-six financial institutions in thirty-seven countries, including Citigroup, JPMorgan Chase, and Wells Fargo. The principles mandate, among other things, a "baseline of social and environmental conditions," the "consideration of feasible environmentally and socially preferable alternatives," and the "protection and conservation of biodiversity . . . including endangered species and sensitive ecosystems." Because most big projects like Ambatovy draw on financing from global banks, financiers hold extraordinary power to attach conditions to their funding, shaping what mining projects look like.

The Equator Principles are not, in origin, moral statements. They are a way of managing risk. That the Equator Principles have become nearly ubiquitous is a reflection of how disruptive and expensive protests near a mine site can be and the extent to which consumer campaigns damage banks' reputations. They are the capitalist's response to powerful outcry.

If Ambatovy's report looked better than I expected, it seemed to come from these overlapping obligations, marks of a shifting industry. To help Madagascar harness more of the economic potential of its resources, Ambatovy was opening a refinery on the coast, shipping value-added products—nickel and cobalt briquettes—rather than raw ore to be processed elsewhere. They were opening training centers to upskill Malagasy workers so they could take jobs in welding, electricity, piping, and instrumentation. They'd committed to buying food from local producers for the cafeteria and having their uniforms made and repaired by Malagasy workers. An uptick in HIV occurred in many boomtowns, and Ambatovy frontloaded the problem with peer education training programs and easily available condoms. There were frog breeding centers intended to keep rare species alive until the land could be put back together. There were hectares of forest set aside for conservation, to offset their mining activity.

Scrolling through the report, I kept telling myself: no company is going to put out a report focusing on what is wrong. The report is not the same as what is happening on the ground. And besides, the mine has only just started production.

I knew in my body that the worst-case scenarios for mining were important. And yet here was my prayer: that maybe a mining project could nourish the people it came to rather than leave a trail of detritus. That a device we called lifesaving could enhance human lives all the way through its supply chain, long before it landed in a chest pocket.

From that moment, ten months of grant applications (and rejections) unfolded, overlapping with a few months of fevered crowdfunding.

Finally: I was going to see it for myself.

From the dripping jungle, Anja and I crested uphill, over some lip, and the trees fell away. We drove into the red heart of the mountain. We emerged into the valley of ore. What would have been the insides of a mountain gaped open, with lines of trucks crawling its edges.

On the ridges flanking the pit, some of the jungle was jungle. Some of the jungle was bones. We drove past stands of dense growth, vined, and we drove past gray, ghostly ridges where the trunks had been taken. Stumps one foot tall, two feet tall had been left, the lop not always clean. At the road cuts, I could see the mat of roots, feet-deep, tangled. I saw where the black topsoil, an eon of jungle, turned to red. The roots appeared not to know their trees were gone. They had not yet had time to dry out, to shrivel, to rot into the earth.

A village, too, had been disappeared from this mine site, twenty-nine households moved elsewhere: the place once called Berano.

At the dozer edge, one mat of roots sat tipped up on end. "The roots will be compost," Anja told me, following my gaze. "We will need lots of compost." She was talking about reclamation, which she called restoration. For ten years this forest crawled with biologists inventorying species, establishing an amphibian breeding center, identifying scraps of azonal forest to leave intact. They hoped that the conservation buffer zone—forest typical for this area, located around the rim of the deposit—would hold species like a vault.

Madagascar is one of the few nations in the world where the real GDP per capita was lower in 2010 than it was in 1970; only the Democratic Republic of the Congo and Liberia, which suffered civil war, experienced more economic decline over that forty-year period.

In Madagascar's case, political crises in 2002 and 2009, in combination with repeated droughts, cyclones, and plagues, strained a country that struggled to attract investment from abroad because of its underdeveloped infrastructure. As of 2012, more than three-quarters of the population lived in extreme poverty. And yet it was also known for its biodiversity. Originally part of the supercontinent Gondwana, the island first broke away from Africa and then, eighty-eight million years ago, found itself left behind when India drifted north. The asteroid that hit the earth approximately sixty-five million years ago, marking the end of the dinosaurs' reign, seems also to have extinguished most animals on land. Madagascar's endemic species are thought to have evolved from "colonization events," in which tangles of vegetation broke off the Mozambiquan coast or floated down rivers to the sea and crossed the Mozambique Channel—a journey of around thirty days. This "rafting" favored animals that could cling to vegetation; the four mammalian groups that made it to Madagascar all live partially in trees, and reptiles who cannot bear salt water on their skin are rare in Madagascar.

Here, then, was the gamble: that the big investment of an extraction project could buoy the country's economy without destroying what was arguably its richest resource.

I was thinking about the difference between those words. A jungle might be reclaimed. But I could not imagine it restored.

The day before I flew to Madagascar, I found myself in the wide mouth of an Apple store in the largest mall in Illinois, twenty minutes from my parents' house. All those years I'd continued to use the same battered 2004-model flip phone, occasionally breaking one and ordering another online. By then I had received a significant number of garbled texts. Images arrived as a question mark. Uncertain of how I wanted to record interviews on the trip, unclear whether hauling my heavy laptop made sense, and in possession of a tiny, recently shattered iPod, I was considering whether I should purchase new technology: a new iPod, or maybe an iPad, or—at the Verizon store down the hallway—an iPhone with my long-overdue upgrade.

In the Apple store, an army of blue-shirted professionals gestured at slim metal laptops on long white counters. The other people in the room looked like they were having fun, shiny paper bags tucked over their wrists, their children clenching cinnamon pretzel samples and not looking where they were going. I felt a heat rise into my face, a scrambled sort of confusion, as a very nice man walked me through the latest generation of iPod touches, which he boasted could do everything an iPhone could do except call. I realized I hadn't slept a full night, in my preparations, in a very long time. From a reporting perspective, it made the most sense to get an iPhone, so I could swap my SIM card for one that would work in Madagascar. And yet as I stood in the Apple store, I suddenly became overwhelmed by the amount of microelectronics in the room, found myself picturing the gleaming insides of each computer, each tablet, each phone checked by customers waiting in line. The cheerful way people around me swapped out electronics hardly a few years old seemed all at once delusional, even nauseating. I set my flip phone and my spider-webbed, slightly spastic, completely full 2010 iPod on the table and tried to square the factors at hand. Would I be that much safer in my traveling if I got an iPhone? By how much? What was that potential safety worth?

And then I laughed, a bark. For wasn't this, after all, the question at hand?

In the end, confused and frustrated and embarrassed, I burst into tears, and my parents and I left. I could make the decision according to what felt like everyone else's criteria—or I could make the decision in a way that reflected my work, this long line of questioning around my own defibrillator. That afternoon I wished furiously that I could just forget what a thing was made of. We live according to the rules of the world we inhabit. Yet it seemed absurd to me that my trip to the African continent to understand what it takes to make microelectronics could get wound up in an argument for purchasing more of them.

I was implicated—we all were—but that day, at least, I couldn't say yes.

Later that night, at a wine bar in downtown Arlington Heights, my mother told me about an article she'd read in the SADS newsletter, about a family in which the older two kids died nine years apart and then the third went into cardiac arrest and made it. Only then were doctors able to look at her EKG and figure out what had killed the other two.

"Three out of three," she said, her hand resting lightly on her glass of Zinfandel. "And two of them dead. So whatever you find on your journey," she said, "it's okay to have it in there. It's okay to get the battery changed." She nodded and nodded, her eyebrows up, looking me dead in the face. She was trying to be firm. What I heard was pleading.

The Ore Preparation Plant sat at the very top of the Ambatovy mine holding, nearly 3,300 feet above sea level. When the big beds of the articulated trucks dumped the ore, it got filtered through a screen that took out the big rocks and roots. What remained went up a conveyor belt and got sprayed with water to separate dust from rock. The rocks were spit out into a pile outside to be used in road maintenance; it was the dust the company wanted. In two cylinders with turning blades, the dust was combined with flocculents, thickening agents. The slurry needed a precise consistency in order to slide down the pipeline, which stretched more than two hundred kilometers from this ridge to the processing plant in Toamasina, by the sea. The pipe held a precise downward tilt, with no additional pumps after its beginnings here in the highlands.

The slurry was sent only when requested by the refinery, which paid attention to prices and orders. It took thirty-six hours for the slurry to pass those 22,000 lengths of pipe, to pass through mountains and beneath rivers. When it reached the refinery, it spouted into a tank, the solids left to settle. When the prices were low, they didn't send it: slurry remained in a tank at the Ore Preparation Plant, poised, waiting. The company stockpiled the low-grade ore and ran the highest-quality first, to pay back investors faster. They processed just enough to pay their bills when prices were low.

There was no dynamite, but the sound of rocks cascading, thudding—the metal screech of machinery—was everywhere.

At the refinery in Toamasina, too, the villages had been removed:

off the plant site and off the tailings field. To make metal one must dismantle houses of wood and build new ones from concrete, with tin roofs and clean beige paint, according to the World Bank's standards on involuntary resettlement and the International Finance Corporation's guidelines for resettlement action plans. In the new villages, locals had access to a school, a health center, and arable land. I hadn't gone to see them; I had bungled the logistics. But in Toamasina I had ridden Ambatovy's shuttle past the places where daily village life used to unfold, now cluttered with ramps, storage tanks, lattices of metal, steaming stacks, fire, and lights. The refinery was visible from miles south as you came up from Brickaville.

Here the toxic alchemy of making nickel and cobalt briquettes began, the dissolution and decanting, the heating and spinning. A rock is a complicated thing; a crushed rock is full of surprises, compounds clinging to one another that must be separated. Some of the rock was worthless, Material of No Economic Value piped away to sit forever in the tailings field. Or as long as it remained untouched by wave, by storm, by wind. Where before there lay the tombs of humans—dug up and moved during resettlement—there now stretched a graveyard for mountains.

Think of the old alchemists, leaned over the flame, trying to make gold from base metals. At Ambatovy the work was clearer, the metals they forged purer. The refinery separated out residual iron, aluminum, copper, and silica through filtration, sedimentation, and extraction with organic solvents. Do not mistake this word *organic*: this was not a solution of water and vinegar from your grandmother's kitchen. *Solvent,* from the Latin *solvō,* meaning, *I loosen, I untie, I solve*; solvents dissolve other things. Mixed with a solvent, gases or solids become solutions; the amount dissolved dictates the strength of the solution. Organic solvents, these powerful unmakers, are volatile, highly flammable. Solvent vapors, exposed to air, can explode.

Solvents are known carcinogens, neurotoxins, reproductive-system hazards. Spills and leaks would filter down through the ground, contaminate aquifers, establish long plumes, and trash human organs.

I learned: this is how we make metal. This is what it means to make a briquette of cobalt, of nickel. To pack it in a drum, to send it by train to the port, to ship it across the Indian Ocean to Asia.

The alchemy of making pure metal is one of taking the world apart.

On the day before the mine tour, I'd met a driver in a rental-car lot at dawn in the port town of Toamasina. We'd followed Route Nationale 2 south through the coastal plains, where gently rolling grasses shone gold in the morning light. Then the highway veered west, and the mountains rose before us, the road tightening into hairpin turns as it wound its way up the 1,640-foot escarpment of the Malagasy highlands. The low clouds of the jungle darkened the sky; then came the first windshield strikes of rain.

Years earlier, I'd been a senior sociology major haunting the cowboy bars and coffee shops of Pinedale, Wyoming, trying to understand how the natural gas boom unfolding there—then the largest in the United States—was changing people's relationships to their homes. A new technology called hydraulic fracturing—"fracking"—had made it possible to extract natural gas from extremely tight sand formations, and so into the tiny town of Pinedale descended thousands of workers who lived in the new hotels springing up or in "man camps" at the edge of town. Just west of Pinedale lay the Wyoming Range, the chain of mountains that had brought me to myself on those high school backpacking trips—and for this reason, my thesis project was personal. Because the Range, too, was vulnerable to drilling as a result of Bush administration–era policies, I wanted to understand what it looked like on the other side of losing what you loved. I wanted to know why some people could take it all in stride—the trucks firing back and forth through town, the influx of men, the blazing lights that blotted out the stars, the sudden problems with air quality, the drilling rigs set up in critical mule deer, pronghorn, and sage grouse habitat—while some of us went to pieces, threatened at our very core by the changes in the place we loved.

It was Pinedale I couldn't stop thinking of as I arrived in Moramanga, another boomtown swollen with migrants in search of work, where on the edge of town those who'd landed coveted mining jobs felled trees and built two-story houses. In Moramanga, the population had been around 37,000 in 2007; by my visit in 2014, it had ballooned to near 50,000. Trash services couldn't keep up with the influx. Traffic jammed on the road. On the highway huge trucks carrying shipping crates from Asia tipped dangerously over the middle line.

In Moramanga, I had a room at the Bezanozano, the big Chinese hotel with the chipping façade built for the mining company's executives when they came to town. As my ears, I'd hired the general manager of the hotel, a slender man named Olive. Olive wanted to be a Baptist missionary someday, which explained why his English was so good in a country where bilingual speakers generally knew Malagasy and French. Because I'd reported only a few stories in the States before I hopped a plane to the Red Island, it hadn't occurred to me to choose a mine in a former British colony, where every kid in a school uniform I met in the street would want to practice their English, as I'd experienced in Sierra Leone. Nor had I ever heard of "fixers"—the trusted locals journalists hire to help them set up the right interviews, get around, navigate regional politics, and interpret the language. My best idea was to e-mail the fanciest hotel in town, the one most likely to anticipate the needs of Americans.

Olive liked the American accent, and he liked America. On the day I checked into the hotel, he wore a Phoenix Suns jersey. He spoke with his eyes opened wide, nodding after each thing he said, adding, "Yes, yes," emphatically, as though I did not believe him.

Knowing that Olive was the general manager, I assumed he was responsible for the gold-edged *Testamenta Vaovao* in my nightstand drawer.

Half a block from my hotel was the place called the T: where the highway from the capital met the road to the coast. Over the course of three days people would tell me, again and again, about the women who worked the T. And should I have been surprised? It was a boom-town; this was what happened when a certain type of man got money. When Olive took me to visit his extended family one afternoon, they clustered on the sofas in the front room of their house to tell me about the girls, some just sixteen, who'd dropped out of school to sell sex. Neighbors hung in the open front window, listening, staring at the *vazaha,* white girl. Olive's family members were schoolteachers, which is why they knew the problem intimately: the money was too good. In Moramanga, there wasn't much work for people with secondary degrees; you had to go to the capital to continue on to university, and then maybe you could come back. These girls, they made 15,000–80,000 ariary a night selling sex: the equivalent of $5.70 to $30.42.

Which was worth it; food had become so expensive since the mine went in. Now there were migrants buying food and Ambatovy buying for their cafeteria in the local market—wiping out stand after stand, driving up the prices.

The men who visited the sex workers were married, Olive's family told me. They had money because of their jobs at the mine. Somehow in Olive's living room I couldn't stop thinking of the mitigation report. I'd been so impressed. Later, I looked up the figures. By the time I spoke with Olive's family against the din of downtown Moramanga, Ambatovy's fifty-three peer educators had spoken to more than three thousand employees about HIV prevention and performed more than two thousand HIV tests.

It was, in a sense, still impressive. Despite workers arriving in Moramanga from across the country, from other parts of the world, there had been no HIV epidemic. Yet I was beginning to sense a more subterranean level of social problems, those it would be hard to touch with a program because they came about through a particular kind of free will, people adjusting to the world they lived in. In general, I honored people's ability to make a living however they could; in particular, I understood what it meant for young girls to drop out of school in favor of turning tricks. Should I consider these decisions, the way a person hustled food onto the table, as an extended consequence of the metal in my body? That this place now bred a certain set of conditions it hadn't before? Boomtowns and sex work have long gone hand in hand. So, too, the grief and disorientation of living in a place as it changes.

Yet all over the world we use our bodies as we can, to make it through another day.

Olive and I circled the mine. Or we circled its stories, as best we could, over the course of the three days I had in Moramanga.

In a hair salon, the coiffeur told us the mine hadn't been good for the town, even though she did more hair now. In the market, beside heaping platforms of tomatoes and jute sacks of beans, a vendor in a red wrap skirt told us about the inflation, about how business had spiked and then dropped. In the office of the first assistant to the mayor of Moramanga Commune, an Ambatovy calendar hung on the wall, but the administrator was stern in his admonishments that the company should employ local businesses as its subcontractors rather than hiring cheaper teams from abroad. Fidgeting with the collar of his gray button-up, he told us about the committees that would decide what to do with the money—a new market? schools? roads?—when it finally came through from the Chamber of Mines. Ambatovy had so far been slow to pay, with all of civil society scrambling to make sure accountability measures were in place before the company transferred millions of dollars to the government.

In Ampitambe, one of the small villages near the turnoff to the mine road, we sat with women on long woven mahampy mats. One woman wound mahampy reed into a basket, carefully alternating the strips. The others watched the road, paved by Ambatovy, an exceptionally smooth piece of asphalt for Madagascar. People here were angry, Olive told me. At first, there had been construction jobs that any man could do. But that was over now. An older woman, wearing a brown felt hat and two twisted braids, gestured toward a man who'd walked up, who squatted against a house in a camouflage T-shirt and jeans. "This man wants to be working," Olive translated, "but all the jobs require degrees."

The problem, I knew, was common to industrial mining projects: always the construction boom, followed by the contraction. Technological advancements had turned mining into the work of machines. Once upon a time, having a mine in a community might have offered long-term economic stability; now many of the positions were technical, staffed in this case by engineers and geoscientists flown in from the capital or from Europe, where they'd been trained. Though Ambatovy employed more than 90 percent Malagasy, in a country with eighteen ethnic groups and jobs at such a premium, an out-of-town employee was still often viewed as not native enough.

I'd read that mining in the 1880s often led to innovation through ad hoc problem solving, technologies developing beside the pit that had other applications—things like the steam engine, which enabled much of the furious growth Western countries benefited from during the Industrial Revolution. But discoveries couldn't be made all over again; any innovation in mining now was unlikely to cast echoes into other fields. It wasn't that mining didn't bring growth or opportunity to a place like this; it did. But the doctrine of mining as a game changer seemed to me inflated, tied to a past whose opportunities were not reproducible and to metal markets that were unpredictable.

Perhaps the corporate social responsibility report that had looked so good was just the latest artifact of a powerful mining mythos, the way industrialization captured our hopes and then—to varying degrees—let us down. Madagascar was a latecomer in a globalized world where economic niches had already been carved out. The goods and services needed for this project could be cheaply and easily provided by nonlocals, and as the train lines and ports and roads that brought them in were improved, imports would cheapen, forcing Moramanga vendors, previously isolated, to compete against products from across the globe—the common extractive-industry ill known as Dutch disease. There would be economic growth, yes, but the way it spidered across the economy might be less potent than it seemed.

There were these big ideas, these white papers and books I'd read, these analyses. And then there were the people sitting on the mahampy mat before me in the clear sweet winter sunlight. The little girl running up to me, squealing, running away. The woman with her hair in two neat buns, nursing a baby. A red chicken careening toward us, then darting away.

The people lived down here in the village, Olive said—picking a naked corncob up off the ground, gesturing with it—but they'd always gone into the hills for what they needed. There was land for making rice, land for gathering firewood, land for hunting bush meat. It had always been this way, until it wasn't.

I understood that they knew their land in a way I had never known any place—in a way I couldn't. I was ecologically native to nowhere. A blur of genes from western Europe and Scandinavia, dragged through Tennessee and Texas on one side and straight to Chicagoland on the other, born of strip malls and sledding hills, camped, like my ancestors, on stolen indigenous land. I'd moved every few years to a different patch of earth, inhabited only temporary communities and cosmologies. When I'd interviewed ranchers and farmers outside Pinedale for my sociology thesis, I felt a kind of ache under my breast-bone at the way they talked about the land: bends in the rivers they knew by heart, the way the moose browsed in the haystacks on winter mornings. I'd had the sense then that I was behind, that it would take half a lifetime to begin to know those aspen and pine forests as deeply as I craved—and look how that had turned out.

I carried an old scar tissue around land: I was used to seeing it cleaved into pieces, some of it "sacrificed" to industry, some of it "saved." In Ampitambe, the wounds were still fresh, the construct foreign.

The mining project took all they had, Olive said. The government in Antananarivo gave permission without consulting them. The most fertile land was gone. They were paid, but not much—and unlike land, money went quickly.

Everyone used to work planting, the women told us, their faces tired, but this could no longer be. There was a job-skills training program no one from this village was chosen for—because of corruption, the women said. Though it was true that Ambatovy built a clinic, it only opened twice a week, and then only to fifteen or twenty people. And villagers wanted the school to no longer require fees, because they could not afford to pay them—not even in rice, now that they did not have fields.

At the very least, they thought, more people from their village should be hired.

One part of the forest still existed, but it was the conservation buffer zone. Even what was not dug up was off-limits. People had been arrested for going back. One man died after his time in prison, and the company took out a half-page ad in the country's major news-papers to clarify that his death was unrelated to his incarceration. He died neither in prison nor from an obviously related ailment, it said. The man and his companions, the company pointed out, had broken the law by crossing into the mining area.

In Vohitranivona, a village tucked off the road to the mine, a girl in a crisp white T-shirt and jeans, sitting on a long mahampy mat, shrugged at me. She had a wide, open face and a short braid. Since Ambatovy had been there, she said, life had become very good for her. It had become easy to find money. Everyone had built a house. It was very safe there, with the new police station Ambatovy built. There were new water pumps, occasionally broken, but generally very good. Up the street we saw concrete house after concrete house, colorfully painted, with beautiful porches and balconies.

A quarter mile away in Ambohinierenana, at dusk, the air smelled of smoke, sweat. People were pissed. One of the *tangalamena*—or elders—stood with me in the middle of a rapidly growing crowd. He spoke for the village, and as he did, people crowed, pitched forward, hollered out. The kids jostled at my feet, more of them all the time, the village emptying into the square. These people had lost access to the forest. But Ambatovy did not build them clean water pumps, as it had for the residents of Vohitranivona. The people had to share clinic time. No one from this village got a job at the mine.

"The land can feed them during their entire life," Olive said. "But not the money."

The *tangalamena,* in a clean blue button-up, told us the company brought them saplings to take care of. The company said it would buy them back in three years. "But three years is too long to wait to feed the family," said the elder. So the village sold the saplings as wood in Moramanga. The company also asked them to form a community association, to grow food crops the company could buy. Despite the company's dedication to sourcing food locally, to strengthening the economy with its enormous purchasing power, it was hard to find a reliable supply. It fed one thousand employees and three hundred sub-contractors lunch at the mine site every day of the week. Community associations, growing crops to sell the company—this was not interest-ing to the villagers, Olive told me. They wanted their normal life back. "They have been here a long time. They cannot leave their own town."

In the golden light of dusk the houses lining the square showed their wooden ribs, mud crumbling off their walls. I looked down. Nearly all the people clustered around me stood barefoot on the packed earth. I felt all of a sudden the weight of these stories, of the loss they were living. I had been drawn to Madagascar by complicity—the metal in my body making me, by some measure, to blame for the grief around me. To the world of the internet these people did not exist, except as the mining company chose to portray them, and in this moment I too became the problematic custodian of their stories— capable of asking the wrong things, of misunderstanding, of bungling the translations. It was easy to think the power I held, as a white American who might someday be handed the microphone, could be used in their service, and yet that wasn't how relationships of power usually played out. Across the road in Vohitranivona sat the artifacts of good intentions like mine, emblazoned with a logo. Some of the people drank cold water pumped from a well. Here, it seemed, there lived only heartbreak.

"They cannot say Ambatovy did not do anything," Olive said, spreading his hands, "but they want more compared to the land they lost."

"You can never, ever please everyone," Anja said at the end of our mine tour, on the way down the hill, as we passed the security check-point, where men in safety vests smiled and waved us through. What she meant was that the people in the villages thought there must be a conspiracy if jobs existed and they did not get them. She meant there were many, many thousands of people in all these villages and Moramanga, and they could not all have jobs at the mine. Only twenty-one of the one thousand employees at the pit, she said, were expatriates. She told me that although the company ran technical training programs, offered scholarships, built wells and hospitals and schools, taught people to make foie gras to sell to restaurants that cater to the French, partnered with the government on major infrastructure projects, and reached out to villages through a grievance program— there was no way to reach everyone. The gestures always fell short.

"We are not a government," she said. "We do what we can, but we have to get nickel and cobalt out of the ground."

On my last morning in Moramanga, rain dumped from the sky. I packed my bags and went seventeen miles down the highway to Andasibe, a village bordering Andasibe-Mantadia National Park, to talk to the biologists who'd inventoried species before the mine went in, who now ran the amphibian breeding center.

By noon, it had become my birthday on the other side of the world. I was twenty-nine. At the Vakona Forest Lodge down the road, I drank a cold glass of white wine, ordered a bowl of tomato soup, and ate a chocolate lava cake roll. Then I walked down the hill to meet the guide who would take me to Lemur Island.

The guide pushed a few bananas into my hands and peeled one more. "Put some in your pockets," he told me. "Now give me your camera."

"What?" I said, and then I understood: lemurs were landing on my head, leaping onto my shoulders, swinging from the trees, and falling in blurs. They perched on my neck and arms, angling to nab the smeary banana bits between my fingers. It went without saying that this was not best practice; I was feeding lemurs rescued from the captive animal trade the equivalent of candy, an empty treat of tourism. Yet from the moment they arrived I felt only joy, wild laughter bubbling up, as the silky fur of a black-and-white ruffed lemur pressed into my forehead, as the tiny hands of brown lemurs combed through my hair, as their animate, intelligent faces looked into mine.

We boarded a canoe and set off down the brown river, ducking thick vines, spatters of rain shaking down off high foliage. Where we climbed back ashore, a fluffy diademed sifaka with a golden belly perched across from me, trembling, nervous. I extended my hand to her, spoke softly, waited minutes. Finally she reached out. She placed her hand on my hand, as though to steady it. Her touch was leathery and cool. Slowly she leaned forward, eyes trained on mine, to lick the banana from my fingers. The guide's face a map of surprise: "I've never seen that one eat from anyone's hand before." The lemur did it again, quietly holding my hand, her little opposable thumb curled around my outstretched palm, leaning close. The soft scratch of her tongue on my fingers. My heart swelling. Her dark eyes testing me.

Later, after the final stop—where ring-tailed lemurs ran circles around my body—it would be the trembling sifaka I thought of as I climbed the hill back to where my driver napped. How the biologists had charted the lemur hollows and knocked. How they'd built those bridges from tree to tree, to steer lemurs deeper into what forest remained. How the sifaka had looked at me cautiously, to see whether I was worthy of trust.

Out of Andasibe, the road twisted steeply downhill. Somewhere to the left of me, I knew, that pipeline punctured the mountains; once in a while, a slurry rushed down it. Now for the first time I saw it: all the red hillsides. Hillsides knit with elaborate maps of trees, knots of roots, bright flowers and quiet animals. I thought of Heidegger in "The Question Concerning Technology," his conclusion that modern technology had fundamentally altered the nature of the earth: "The earth now reveals itself as a coal mining district, the soil as a mineral deposit. The field that the peasant formerly cultivated and set in order...appears differently than it did when to set in order still meant to take care of and to maintain [rather than driving on to maximum yield at minimum expense]....What the river is now, namely, a water power supplier, derives from out of the essence of the power station....Everywhere everything is ordered to stand by, to be immediately at hand, indeed to stand there just so that it may be on call for a further ordering."

It was likely these hillsides contained only low concentrations of metal, if any at all, and yet to see the color there beneath so much life—so much overburden—stole my breath. That the world could be so dismantled for the right price. That it was no longer earth but ore. That I had told a doctor yes, to put the metal inside me.

I was supposed to believe my own life worth all this.

"No one is thinking about the ants," the biologist Jean-Noël Ndriamiary had quietly said during our interview that morning, as we sat together in the gently shifting forest. He meant that an intact ecosystem is too complicated to save piecemeal; we don't even know what all the pieces are.

A colony of ants is not a lemur, capable of looking a human in the eye. Yet in the biologist I detected grief. I could not forget now that every being in the ecosystem was ensouled and essential, the coppery trampled plants and the singing frogs and all the species of insects we hadn't yet named.

At night, the smell there was always one of beautiful, burning trees.

CHAPTER 6

Maroseranana, Madagascar
2014

By the time we crossed past the boundary of the Conservation International area, where people weren't supposed to cut trees, a steady downpour had settled over the jungle. For hours the forest had been slowly expanding as I followed my guide, Stephan, and interpreter, Mirielle, from sunny river valleys onto the long, muscular shoulder of a mountain, the wooden houses and snack shops growing sparse. Then the trail went to orange ooze. Mirielle and Stephan, walking in rubber sandals, gave up on the drier edges of the trail and marched instead straight into the muck.

Seventy kilometers from here, as the bird flew, stretched the giant gash of the Ambatovy mine. That swath of jungle had been just like this one, except for its economically recoverable nickel and cobalt—and because that jungle was coming down, this one must stay. This was the "mitigation hierarchy" required by the Business and Biodiversity Offsets Programme. In theory, by carefully measuring its negative impacts and "ecosystem enhancements," a company like Ambatovy could break even, achieving a standard of "no net loss." Only here, in the rainforest called Ankerana—a stretch recently incorporated into the internationally heralded Ankeniheny-Zahamena Corridor (CAZ)—it was the people themselves who had been deemed a threat to the forest. Their age-old practice of *tavy*, clearing forest with fire in order to plant rice on ash-fertile ground, combined with population growth, had put pressure on dwindling patches of forest, especially as climate change led to bigger storms and droughts, disrupting agriculture. The *tavy* rotations left land fallow for fewer years than they had in the past, which meant land was less productive, which meant more of it had to be cleared to keep up with the community's needs. And while population growth can sometimes drive increased efficiency in agriculture, for the Malagasy of the eastern rainforests, the process of *tavy* was as much a ritual that honored their ancestors as it was either a commercial or subsistence activity.

Before we set off from Stephan's home in Anivorano—hoping to talk to the elders of a village perched on the edge of the offset—it had never occurred to me that a biodiversity offset could be morally problematic. That a mining company would be forced to make up for the land it wrecked seemed a just thing; standards such as the Equator Principles—if actually followed—seemed like examples of a system finally righting its own errors. And yet the very concept of a conservation offset was predicated on the Western ideal of empty land, the idea that humans are foreigners to forests and not themselves indelible parts of ecosystems. While it was true that Madagascar's diverse species were increasingly under pressure—and that some of that pressure came from humans—I was learning that human rights cannot be untangled from land rights. Here, to offset one injury meant creating another: displacing not only humans and their livelihoods but also their entire cosmology. Stephan—a tall export-crop farmer and part-time guide with a hooked nose and ears that stuck out—was taking us to Maroseranana, another community that had lost access to the forest where they'd long hunted and gathered. Yet here the loss occurred for the opposite reason: the land would be set aside rather than taken apart.

The way to Maroseranana was a footpath that wound seventeen miles from village to village, crossing through their centers, where wood houses on stilts fanned out over hardened ground. In the largest of the villages, some of the buildings stood two stories tall, each with a tin roof and a long porch above the road and a bright coat of paint. In the smaller villages the homes were woven from strips of bamboo and ravinala. On long wood tables beside them, women sold dried fish like flat disks, shriveled and swirling with flies, while flocks of skinny chickens ducked and darted beneath their feet. We passed zebu, bony humpbacked longhorn cattle, who sprang suddenly into mating on the road beside us, a boy jumping into the herd to whip them onward with a slender stick. We passed broad brown rivers and old cemeteries. We passed a man standing on a bamboo raft piled high with bananas, negotiating whitewater rapids with a pole. We walked through rice fields gleaming bright green beneath a cover of rain, and through thick forest humming with bugs and birdcall. Slipping by on the trail were porters: shirtless men climbing the mountain in stained shorts and ball caps, each with a fat green bamboo pole balanced on either shoulder. The poles were longer than the men were tall and thick as their legs, and on each end hung plastic crates full of empty Three Horses beer bottles for refill in the city, lashed to empty gas canisters. Into this country went only human legs, the skinny zebu, and the occasional motorbike. To see what must be carried out, to see what must be carried in—to see the legs, shining with muscle, that walked back and forth for a living in the mud, barefoot or wearing jelly shoes—stunned me. The men chewed chunks of sugarcane as they passed, spitting the fibers on the road.

The night before, I'd lain in bed in Fetraomby—another village on the path—miserable and feeling guilty for being miserable. The blanket on the bed was wet, left precisely in the place where the tin-and-thatch roof dripped onto the bed when it rained. The smell of mold overwhelmed; the night was cold without a cover. However I'd romanticized this form of reporting when I chose to go, it trafficked in spikes of joy and jags of despair. I was rapidly discovering the limits of Mirielle's English—something I hadn't known how to test—and so carried the loneliness of being unable to enter the worlds of those around me. At dusk in the wood-framed shops, kids had twirled on the posts of the storefronts, candlelight glanced off the faces of pretty women, a man danced barefoot with a square package he'd received. I could only imagine their worlds; I could not overhear. In the version of this journey I carried in my head before setting out, I'd assumed I'd be able to connect with individuals, to flesh out the calculus of what it took to make a defibrillator, to arrive at conclusions about whether, when my battery buzzed low, I should get another one. Yet at night, in bed, finding answers felt like a vision that could slip away into frustration, and it terrified me. It wasn't just eleven thousand miles that separated me from these people. It was also language and culture, skin color and economics. As I lay in bed, a cold fear filled my body: that it had been a waste to send me here. The technology in my chest remained invisible and untranslatable to everyone I met.

To ask what it took to make a defibrillator—and whether it was worth it—was in some way an attempt to put a finger on the scale. The quest to understand how my life was connected to others' offered a sort of accountability, and thus a salve to my guilt. It gave my life a brighter purpose. But if asking the question might make my own life closer to "worth it," this could only work—I thought furiously—if I nailed the interviews, if I noticed the essential details, if I understood people. If I could see the truth at the center of things, and tell the story that mattered. It could only work if I did it *right*.

On the road to Maroseranana, we walked mile after mile soaked with sweat and rain, slipping in calf-deep ooze, my raincoat sopping all the way through and my hip beginning to tweak, until finally we slid and sloshed down the arm of the mountain and turned a corner to see, out of nowhere, a clean white cloth banner pulled taut above the road: TONGASOA ETO MAROSERANANA. Welcome to Maroseranana.

In the lower right-hand corner, the logo of the mining company.

It was only another minute to the company's complex, perched on the outskirts of town. The concrete building was a crisp and unsullied yellow, with firmly shuttered windows and flowering shrubbery at the front door. A satellite dish angled off its roof. When Mirielle told me we were staying there—moving toward a green row of guesthouses—I laughed out loud. Of course. The mining project I'd come to scrutinize would be, unbeknownst to them, housing me. I laughed at the brand-new bunk beds with bright sheets and new mosquito nets. I laughed at the flat-screen TV locked in a cabinet next to our dinner table, at the empty bottle of J&B Scotch beside it. I laughed—after days of pooping in bamboo stalls roiling with maggots and cockroaches—to see the upright porcelain toilet, which automatically discharged some kind of cleaning liquid into itself. I had taken a lurching bus from the capital to the coast, caught a ride in a packed and sputtering car up a washboard road, ridden pillion on a motorbike in the mud, and walked seventeen miles into the jungle in the rain only to find myself, a white Westerner, afforded a fine toilet and a stiff drink. Of course it was the property of a mining company. Their display of wealth, gaudy in the context of these villages, at that moment filled me with relief. It was 2:00 p.m. but felt like 4:00—my legs were collapsing under me—and so I did the only thing you would expect of a white American in a jungle: I ate a giant spoonful of Nutella, stripped to my underwear, and climbed into bed.

In the morning we ate mufugas—fluffy, oily little disks of rice flour with pockets of sweetness—and drank a dark, complex coffee. Then the three of us walked up the muddy road from the compound into the village, past the sheet-metal church with a pair of zebu horns hung over its door, past the plant nursery labeled with the mining company's logo, past wooden homes on stilts. The sun was out. Clotheslines hung bright with color.

The president of Maroseranana was happy to see us. After talking briefly with Stephan, he leaned toward me, thrusting his hand out. Then he took off down the block, ducking in and out of wooden storefronts, to collect the *tangalamena*, the town's council of elders. In his white T-shirt, blue athletic shorts, and salmon-colored flip-flops, he looked more like a coach gathering players for a game. "A long time he has wanted people to ask questions about Ambatovy," Mirielle said, nodding her cornrowed head. The president flashed a big white smile at us each time he passed.

The Maroseranana administrative building was a wooden structure raised up on a concrete foundation with a sheet-metal roof and chipping yellow paint. Inside its doorway, two typewriters sat out on a water-damaged wooden table, and I thought of the desktop computers and satellite dish down the street.

The mining company had established the Maroseranana field office to attend to the problem of providing alternative livelihoods. As I had felt with my own sore, muddied body, there wasn't much choice in the way people lived back here; they were simply too far from the nearest economic centers to benefit from opportunities beyond subsistence agriculture. They were dependent on the rice crop the way their parents and grandparents had been. Selling bananas to a larger market required whitewater-surfing a load downstream before they browned; shipping lychees abroad meant first carrying them over the pass on a bamboo pole. Early in the walk, as Mirielle and I had crossed a broad, flat plain fuzzy with banana groves and grasses, she'd pointed out a brown band of water rolling down its center and turned to me, her eyes glinting. "You know why there are holes?" she said. And before she finished, I saw them and knew: the strange divots on the banks, heaps and mounds of sand with grass growing out their exposed tops. Someone had been panning the stream. If you got sick, Mirielle said, or if you couldn't pay the school fees, or if the crop failed because of cyclones, you could come to get the gold. It wasn't much, just flecks, but it was enough.

Now—in Maroseranana, at least—there would be no panning, no burning, no cutting trees to build houses, no hunting lemur as extra food. The company paid a young man to walk the conservation area every month, 180 kilometers on foot between the five villages that bordered Ankerana, to understand whether people were following the conservation rules. His job was to educate people about what they could eat that didn't require *tavy*. Each of the five villages had a new nursery where they grew seedlings for crops—corn, tomato. The company gave some of the seedlings to children, to teach them to grow them, and paid fifteen to twenty people per village to work in the nursery. There were projects raising fish and pigs and birds and bees. Ambatovy had tried to start a big poultry project—distributing chickens that people could grow for slaughter—but some of the hens they handed out were diseased, and the disease spread to the other chickens, killing them.

The men assembled in the president's office, a blue-and-white room with peeling walls. They sat on wooden benches and stools. They leaned against the doorway. The president carried white plastic chairs over his head into the room. The mayor, wearing an aqua windbreaker and gray suit pants, settled himself at a desk near the front, his fingers threaded together.

We went around the room: The foreman of administration. The number one adviser. A member of the city council. The director of schools. The number two adviser. A man who grew up in Maroseranana but lived in the capital now, working for Airtel, who happened to be back to visit. He haltingly introduced himself in English.

A tiny old man with weathered feet and deep cheekbones, winter cap askew, introduced himself simply, and everyone in the room laughed. "He says he is an old man," Mirielle translated, smiling.

The complaints were these: Ambatovy did not pay the people working for them enough. They did not build them new schools or a new administration building, although they did put a new roof on one of the school buildings. "Ambatovy helps, but with a limit," said Mirielle. People wanted a hospital. People wanted a road from Fetraomby so they could export cassava, lychee, coffee, and banana. "People want more than Ambatovy will give," Mirielle said. "They want things that can benefit the entire community."

One of the unexpected side effects of Ambatovy's presence in town, they told us, was that NGOs no longer came to offer services. Yet Ambatovy did not meet the people's needs. There was no clean water. "There is a big problem if Ambatovy leaves," Mirielle said. "Before, a man plants rice. Now he works for Ambatovy."

"Everyone is asking, 'Why does Ambatovy give to everybody else, but not to me?' In this way, the community is strained," Mirielle said. There was much, it seemed, that had been bearable only as long as it was the same for everyone. What the company brought carried with it hard-to-measure losses.

The men spoke quickly, overlapping, and I struggled to catch who said what, struggled to parse Mirielle's translation before she moved on. *Ambatovy's gifts are not enough for all the people. Why haven't they built the road? Ambatovy is working in the country because of the government but the government isn't looking at things.*

It was a long way to come only to turn around, but by tradition the *tangalamena* spoke for the town, and they had spoken. And so that afternoon we picked our way through the mud, back over the pass to a tiny village called Berapaka, located about halfway through the walk to Stephan's house in Anivorano, where we had begun. In the darkness Berapaka roared with the sounds of yelling children, water hitting the ground, the thump of pestles hulling rice, the rise and fall of humming insects. Smoke from cooking fires seeped out the raffia roofs of the houses. Stars cast a white net in the sky. By flickering kerosene lamp we ate rice and salty hot papaya, a chicken with just shreds of meat on its bones, baby bananas. We drank ranovola, the leftover water from cooking the rice, a bitter, starchy drink.

Late that night, once Mirielle and I were curled into our beds—flat planks with a mattress of stuffed banana leaves and grass, and only a thin sheet—I heard her shift. "Why doesn't Ambatovy give aid to Berapaka?" she asked. And I knew we had both noticed the desperation in this town: the blankets we should have had on the beds that night—given to the villagers by the ecotourism organization that employed Mirielle and Stephan—were gone, sold for extra cash; the children were skinnier, their clothing more tattered. The answers I had for her were too easy: *Berapaka has nothing to do with Ambatovy.* The people here did not lose access to their forests. They did not host an office for the company. They were not resettled by mining. They merely lived in a village through which a few more motorbikes now came and went, on a stretch of mud road that made commerce and the delivery of health care nearly impossible. I had noticed in the meeting with the *tangalamena* the rarity with which the men suggested that anything was the fault of their government; it seemed they'd never expected their government to offer them health care in the first place, or widen and grade their road, even with the taxes and royalties it would receive from Ambatovy.

They expected more from a multinational mining corporation.

Despite running social and environmental programs to manage their material impacts, extraction companies were not fundamentally in the business of improving the human condition, no matter how many smiling children adorned their corporate responsibility reports. They were good at moving and refining rock; their intention was to profit. The products made from this rock, much later, might improve the human condition in places far from here, but their only obligation in this place was to roughly break even, to satisfy their investors and funders and the Malagasy government. And yet Mirielle's observation—*Why doesn't Ambatovy give aid to Berapaka?*—rent open a question that could not be ignored in the context of global inequality, in countries with a poverty rate like this one.

So much of the argument for resource extraction is the "development" it brings. But development doesn't exist in the way we act like it does, as a bright monolithic savior, as the inevitable and seamless outcome of large foreign investment. The rising tide only lifts all boats if policy ensures that it does. In the meantime, there are plenty of accidental ways a mining project can make things worse. Big mining projects tend to strengthen the value of the currency anywhere they unfold, making the host country's exports seem expensive and less attractive on the global marketplace while cheapening imports from elsewhere, cratering local manufacturing and agriculture. The larger the proportion of a country's money from natural resources, the less democratic that country tends to be; leaders who aren't dependent on their tax base don't need to earn popular approval, and they have more reason and ability to stay in power with such an asset to draw on. Foreign actors might notice incentive to prop them up, if it buys access to the "honey pot"; meanwhile, political adversaries might find payoff in a violent coup.

The hope that resource extraction will better the lives of ordinary people isn't all hollow—nations can, as if by magic trick, turn these one-time-only forms of capital into resources that seed other industries, investing in their citizens in ways that resonate long after the rock is gone. Viewed in its best light, the conservation offset bordering Maroseranana was such an investment, preserving the famed species that could someday sustain a steady flow of ecotourists. The question was whether the promise of mining—like that of medical technology—could hold a candle to its unintended consequences. Whatever sustainability Westerners thought we were gaining by cordoning off one forest while destroying another wasn't shared by those who lived nearby.

Loss is not experienced in the "net." Grief is not a mathematical calculation. The improved resources of one community don't offset the need for subsistence in others. Losses are specific and exact, shapes that can be soothed but not replaced by gifts and programs.

Perhaps the source of the heartbreak was this: however much a Western presence in these towns created strife, it also came with a brief bright hope—that someone, at long last, would be accountable for improving their lives.

CHAPTER 7

Boulder, Colorado
2009

A fter the surgery there were two kinds of people: those who had suffered in their bodies, and those whose bodies were invisible to them. The second group would move awkwardly in my presence, would not ask the questions that lingered in the room. They did not understand what it meant to be suddenly old. To fear tripping, to become terrified of ice on the ground, to worry over steep stairwells with slick carpet. To sit long hours with the kind of pain that forever changes the architecture of your body.

In the eyes of the first group were all the answers I needed.

The first thing I remember was pain. Searing, immobilizing pain over my left chest.

And in the haze of it, my mother leaning in: "Oza says it's all taken care of. There won't be a bill."

He had donated his fee. The anesthesiologist had donated his fee. St. Jude Medical had donated the defibrillator.

A pectoral muscle does not have room for a metal box. It must be carved—the "pocket." A defibrillator wire is lowered down a vein. Its tip is sharp: a corkscrew packed with steroid. Twisted, the wire anchors into the heart.

Over the months, scar tissue will grow, fueled by steroid, to hold it still. So it can accurately sense.

But this is months after implantation. In the beginning, there is a corkscrew entering flesh.

The day after surgery a storm blew in, unseasonable. First rain in cold strikes. Then snow, a heavy fluff just in time for hospital release. The fall leaves, just beginning to hit their peak, froze on the trees, then fell, mostly still green, then brown. Overnight, town was transformed: a stillness in the neighborhoods, a slush on the sidewalks. A hazard for a heart surgery patient. "Oh great," my mom said.

My mom hadn't made it in time for the surgery. It was Sam who wheeled me down to the cardiac catheterization lab. Beating Heart Bear, riding on my chest, was a hit with the staff.

My mom picked Christine up from class on her way from the airport, and they were there by the time I woke. She told me that when the staff tipped me forward, pressing my back and chest between a mobile X-ray unit, I cried out, and Christine flinched, wept in the hallway, knowing what it felt like.

"What the goddamn is that?" is the second thing I said, according to Christine. The pain pills made me hilarious. Sitting on the edge of my tray was a tiny stuffed lemur with giant eyeballs. My mom and Christine had bought it in the gift shop. "There's always room for more ugly animals," I said. His name would be Lemur. Then: "I'm so fucking hungry."

I came out of surgery already in my sling. The immobilization was to keep my arm from moving in ways that could shift the wire, so freshly placed.

We prayed for close parking spots, and the universe, for once, complied. To walk had become an act of bravery, requiring the type of reserve and composure once reserved for mountain trips. One step after another. Take the time it takes.

* * *

My body became a stranger to me. My very body language shifting in ways that would never reverse. One cannot—with a row of staples and a new lump of metal lodged beneath the skin—hold one's shoulders back. Any restriction of movement like this rapidly leads to degeneration in the muscles, even changes to the mechanical properties of the spine, shifts in the tissues that are hard to walk back. Wearing a sling meant I cradled my left arm upward, protectively, curling my left shoulder in; it meant I could not sleep on my belly or side. Sometimes, long after, I would find myself holding my left arm in this position, close to the body at a diagonal, the ICD resting inside my palm. When I caught myself doing it, I sometimes felt obscene, like the act was akin to squeezing my own breast in public, but the hand, of course, was visibly higher than that and not moving. I was not one of the patients with "twiddler's syndrome," in which a person manipulates the device through the skin, or "reel syndrome," in which she rotates it. No, my hand was just waiting, a shield of sorts. It was the stabilizer I needed in the car, where every bump in the road made the ICD bump inside my body. It was the cushion I needed when the seat-belt strap pulled uncomfortably against my new lump. During sex Sam had to be careful not to lean on me, or if I was on top I needed to remain straight as a soldier, for to lean forward meant using an arm to press against the bed or the wall or the man, and this was too much pectoral, too much pushing on the wound. I did my best to develop core strength.

Our house was still full of stacked boxes. My mom stayed a few days to help me while Sam worked. She helped me put on my clothes. She put plates of food in front of me. She took me to her hotel room at the Holiday Inn and bathed my body in the shallow white tub, my incision taped with plastic.

My mother: whose own mother had been diagnosed with a brain tumor when my mom was just fourteen, who spent her life caretaking through breast cancer and strokes, skin cancer and skull-chiseling surgeries. Who understood what it meant to comfort and assist.

She took me to hair salons, where they gently sat me in the tipping-back chairs to get my head under a faucet. It was the only way not to soak the incision or, worse, to cause the ICD to press against the incision by leaning forward. Sometimes it was five dollars. Sometimes it was free.

My mother braided my hair so I could go more days without it matting.

My mother brought me loose, ugly shirts that didn't require me to move my arms above my head. We slid my arms in slowly, at low angles.

While I rested she helped us unpack. Cleared pathways and organized the kitchen. Sometimes I sat upright in a chair, directing her; she became my arms.

After the staples came Steri-Strips. Dr. Oza told me to let them fall off naturally, but of course I picked at them. "Yeah right they fell off, Kati," Sam said when they were gone, shaking his head.

For the rest of my life I would need device checks: visits to the cardiology office every three months, where a St. Jude technician could drape a wand over my device and download its data through my skin. The wand connected to a St. Jude laptop called a Merlin, and there the tech could see an EKG for any shocks issued, could tell if the device had noticed erratic heartbeats or recorded high heart rates, and their dates and times. "What were you doing at 5:53 p.m. on November thirteenth?" the tech would ask, and I would scrunch my face and pull out my calendar, trying to place the event, which was almost always exercise. Then the tech would test the system by racing my heart—a sudden eerie uptick in heartbeat that felt like nothing so much as a flood of anxiety—then slowing it, a low, stomach-flipping set of palpitations. If all went right, it meant that to the best of our knowledge my wires were still correctly placed, the insulation cover-ing them uncompromised, the ICD itself without defect. It meant that if it needed to, the device was ready to save my life.

On my second weekend after surgery, Sam went climbing in Nevada.

He'd planned the trip two months earlier. I'd been invited, but even then I'd said no for the obvious reasons. Now that the surgery had actually happened, I found myself torn. He had good intentions. But saying no to fun things, outdoor things, made Sam irritable and resentful. Living with me put him on duty as a default. I was unemployed, could not drive, had nowhere to be. I could not even hold a book up; the angle of the motion engaged my pectoral muscles too much. I could not help with the dishes, could not move a cast iron skillet or raise teacups above my head to place them on the shelf. My college friends drove from Denver, from Colorado Springs, to cook for me, to do loads of dishes, to take me for a shampoo, but there was so much else that fell to him. Unlike my mother, he'd never had seriously ill family members or watched someone caretake others, nor had he suffered in his own body in this way. What I wanted him to say was, "Of course I'm not going!" But if he didn't say it himself, I didn't know how to ask him to. I didn't know if it was my right. Didn't know if it would actually help the situation.

The weekend he was gone, Christine came and got my car, with the understanding that she would use it that night, then retrieve me and bathe me in the tub at Alpha Chi Omega the next day. I was greasy, and the apartment on Maxwell had only a shower, something I couldn't believe I'd overlooked in the apartment-choosing process.

Christine never came back for me. All afternoon, as I waited, she didn't respond to my texts. Later that night I got a voice mail from her telling me she'd locked my keys in the car at a liquor store. I was livid, didn't call her back. The one person I thought would understand. The person I needed most.

I would hardly see her until Christmas. Back at our parents' house for the holidays, I confronted her in the kitchen. I told her how poorly she'd treated me that fall, how hurtful it had been. And she cried. She knew she'd been avoiding me—but if she hadn't ever dealt with her own cardiac arrests and surgeries, how could she handle mine?

Kati says I need to say things out loud, she wrote in her journal that night, after we hugged and made up. *It's true. I haven't been dealing well, and it's been affecting other people (like her).* A month later, she reminded herself, *Seeing Kati is a must. She'll be angry for a long time. The truth is, I haven't gotten over the fact that I shouldn't be alive. And I haven't touched the issue in a while because I let routine carry it away.*

She was twenty-one years old.

For Christmas, Sam bought me a train ticket from Chicago to Boston. I'd always wanted to take a long train trip, and he'd invited me to join him at his family's place on Cape Cod for New Year's.

"Remember to ask for help with your bags," my dad cautioned as he dropped me at the train station. "Don't take risks with your wire."

All night the train rumbled through industrial towns across the Midwest. I woke up in New York, a state I'd never been to, and spent the day with my face pressed to the window, watching rivers collect and diverge. The East was a foreign country to me. After what my fall had been, I needed that newness, that open horizon.

The Cape was bitterly cold and wet, the coast soppy with frozen seafoam. Sam took me to his favorite childhood shops, to flooded boardwalks and austere lighthouses and beaches where the sea had swallowed chunks of the land, leaving cliffs laced with dead grasses. We pressed our faces together for warmth. We ducked into steamed-up cafés for pizza and drank rich glasses of red wine. I left him love notes in the wet sand.

All that week, in the flushed glow of exploring with him, I kept thinking, "I want to marry this man."

One night sitting at the kitchen table in his mom's rented condo, we found ourselves talking about how hard things had been. The burden of the dishes, the cleaning I couldn't do because of reaching and turning. The meals he was paying for so that I could be included socially, filling in the edges of the money my dad sent, a situation that caused a flare of anxiety in my belly. More than that, there was the gap of working and not working, his stress, my constant presence and despair—our misaligned sex life, in which I wanted, and he rolled away.

"I don't want to break up with you," he said quietly. "We're not there yet. But."

"I understand," I said. "I know."

"How do you see it?" he asked.

"It feels to me"—I spoke slowly—"like there's a time bomb ticking. It's not in the room yet, but it's looking in the windows."

He was quiet, then nodded. "That sounds exactly right," he said. We both looked toward the glass, toward the dark outside, as though we could see it there. As he took my hand the winter storms were pounding the coast.

CAUSA FINALIS

CHAPTER 8

Boulder, Colorado
2010

On the last good day of our relationship, Sam and I drove out to Pawnee National Grassland, a windswept, hoodoo-filled plain lodged in the armpit between Nebraska and Wyoming. We'd left Boulder in early afternoon, taking back roads he'd never been on, past farm stands and high waves of plains grass. It was the first week of May, and everything was mud from that last spring snow. "I'd never get out here alone," Sam said, and I smiled.

"That's why I'm good for you."

He turned toward the back window, where the Flatirons were sinking into the rest of the Front Range, and stretched out his arm dramatically, grabbing at the air like a child. "But *mountains*!" he said. "Rock climbing!"

"Oh, stop," I said. But I was happy.

I drove these back roads when I tired of the main highway, tracking loops around Boulder County for my new job in the youth services department of a sexual health clinic. In January—after five months of constant applications, and weeks after my temp job at a puzzle factory ended—I'd written a cover letter to the clinic on the thirty-seventh anniversary of *Roe v. Wade*. It was a job I hadn't been able to see myself in (how could I possibly be qualified to work in *health care*, I thought) until, halfway through preparing my materials, the resonance rocked me: this was a feminist organization with the goal of reducing barriers to health care for populations that had been excluded. They offered a sliding payment scale, Spanish translation services, low-cost vasectomies, and a free, confidential clinic for teens—of which I was now the manager.

The clinic booked me all over—from elementary schools to colleges, from halfway houses to teen–parent support groups—to give presentations on contraceptive methods and STI prevention. I liked the faraway stops best because I could zigzag back through these horse pastures, passing slumping barns, catching glints of silver where the irrigation ditches ran.

Out past Greeley the farmland turned to dry grass. Sam and I bumped through the last rail town, with its silent, wind-wrung gas station and faded grain silo. Pumping oil jacks crowned the hills. Sam held my right hand, and I drove with my left.

It was hard to believe that just the day before we'd been fighting bitterly, but it was happening more and more. The spring for me had been a blur of reproductive-health flash cards, packed Teen Clinic nights when I struggled to manage the flow of patients from the front desk, a heavy load of medical and legal protocols to master. An old friend of my dad's—a prominent environmental consultant—had also reached out, looking for a research assistant for his book on corporate water conservation strategies, at $20 an hour. I was exhausted from learning my new job, but this wage was higher than the clinic's, and it was work involving writing. Mostly, the surgery bills had added up— despite Dr. Oza's generous contribution, the donated defibrillator, and the ER financial aid write-offs—to nearly $23,000. I worked weekends and nights to send monthly minimum payments to all the different billing agencies demanding them of me.

At home, I pleaded for alone time after punishing clinic days. Sam, on the other hand, worked long underpaid days from the kitchen table, trying to meet freelancing deadlines and keep a website running. Too often I arrived home to find him frantic with anxiety over all he had to do, wanting me to anchor him. On the weekends, he went to the mountains, but skiing and rock climbing were still too dangerous for the wire slowly attaching to my heart, and now that I managed the Teen Clinic on Saturday afternoons, it was hard to get a day off for other adventures together.

If my life was stabilizing, it still didn't look like it had before. I spent that spring trying to build back my endurance on the steep center trail at Mount Sanitas, running uphill for a minute or two at a time, holding my defibrillator down as it bounced inside my body, as though pledging allegiance to something I wasn't sure I believed in. There was only one sports bra I'd found that cut over at the right angle to help hold the ICD in place, and only if I bought it two sizes too small and wore tight shirts to keep the pressure stiff. My body had swollen over the months of inactivity; I became unrecognizable to myself. Despite my hope that—now having an ICD—someday I could forgo beta-blockers, Dr. Oza was hardly going to let me off them so soon. The beta-blockers held my heart below 130 beats per minute, and a light-headed, throat-clenching sensation took over me when I pushed it. The heart monitor sometimes flashed terrifyingly, leaving me uncertain whether it was the monitor or my heart on the fritz, until finally one day I stopped wearing it, deciding my heart was at most risk from the anxiety of watching it.

The first day I ran the trail all the way to the top, I burst into tears, floating the mile home, exploding through the door to share my news. But Sam didn't seem to see what the big deal was; he was preoccupied. What had happened to my body had happened to mine alone. It wasn't something I could explain to him. I wouldn't understand until much later how this veil between us, thin at first, grew into a thick curtain, a block in our communication that colored everything.

My new job ended one version of our life: the one in which I was always available, the one in which we were moving back to Jackson. The night my new supervisor called me to offer me the job—after we'd rushed out to celebrate with margaritas and chips *con queso* with friends, once we were settled back in bed—Sam got sad. The cabin had been waiting for us in Jackson all this time; we'd need to let go now. We could both picture the valley, moon-white and frozen. We'd left his sailboat in the rickety wooden storage shed and our bed in the house, pushed up against that wall-length window. "Can we wait to call?" he asked. "I'm not ready to give it up just yet." I nestled into his arm. I could almost feel the currents against us, washing us somewhere we hadn't planned on, somewhere we couldn't know.

Now we'd crossed past all the places I knew. The land crisped and widened, the sky a pale blue mouth fixed against the horizon. "It looks like there will be one more road north of here, to take us east if we want to see the buttes," Sam said, holding the map book, his fingers tracing county roads.

"I'm glad we made this work," he added, bumping a kiss against my shoulder. His hair was sweet golden in the afternoon light.

"Me, too," I said.

We'd tried to go to Pawnee a day earlier—on our shared Sunday off. But we'd failed to leave after he lost his to-do list and spent the morning tearing the house apart. "You must have moved it!" he shouted, as I crawled on my belly beneath our futon bed, as I checked under the bookshelf and pink chair again and again, my stomach a hard nut. When he finally found the yellowed Post-it under the nightstand, coated in curls of dust, he slumped back at the kitchen table, and we stared at each other sadly. It was too late to go. But without speaking it aloud, we both knew we needed this trip: a long drive, dirt on our skin, to be together under open sky. Things were bad in our relationship. This daylong adventure was all that was left in our book of tricks.

Sam agreed to leave at noon the next day, after he'd put in most of the East Coast's workday.

We took the turn, crested a hill. Wind farms rose beside us, their long white blades like the arms of strange plains trees. Beyond them, the buttes, a chalky yellow-white, jutted off the grasslands like beehives.

We parked in a dirt lot on the edge of an overlook, beside the brown Forest Service NO CAMPING sign. When we cracked open the door it was windy out, surprisingly cold, and so we ate our snack in the front seat, scooping hot salsa into our mouths with salty chips. Sam gasped dramatically at the heat.

"We're so wimpy," I said, and Sam grinned.

"Are not," he said. "This is fucking hot salsa."

We pulled on our windbreakers, packed water bottles into his small backpack, and set off down the mud trail.

* * *

I still had that headache, the one that had started in the morning, on my slow jog by the creek. It had been a sudden sensation, a wave of pain followed by a weakness in my belly. I'd felt shaky enough to walk home instead of run, letting myself into the house quietly while Sam took a conference call at the kitchen table. I showered, packed the cooler, and prepared a salad for our lunch, drinking as much water as I could, thinking the headache would slip away.

I was chewing a mouthful of greens when I got the first punch of nausea. I put down my fork. Then the headache suddenly became unbearable, crowding in. My skin seized up, hot and sensitive to the touch. I began to shake.

I got up quietly and went to the bathroom, popping three ibuprofen into my palm. I swallowed them down. *It will be fine. It will be fine. It needs to be fine.* I stared at myself in the mirror. *Please.*

"Sam," I said finally, and I told him: the headache, the nausea, the weird sensitivity.

"I don't know what just happened," I said.

He looked at me, concerned, then exasperated. "I don't know what to do with you," he said.

"Me neither," I said miserably, because I had just been *fine,* because I wanted to *go.*

"Just give me a minute," I said, but the shaking was getting worse, my skin felt like hell, the headache so dense and dark I didn't want to keep my eyes open.

"Do I need to take you to the hospital?" I looked at his face, his computer screen still up, our fights so fresh. I felt frantic. No. No hospitals. Was that the only option?

"I don't know," I said. "Let me lie down. Let me take a nap, and we'll see. I bet I'll be fine when the ibuprofen kicks in."

"Are you sure?" he said.

"You keep working," I said, and went into the other room, where I lay shaking until I fell asleep.

When I woke, the world seemed filled with a tentative kind of quiet. The headache was there, but dimmer, more manageable. I felt weak.

But I knew I had to do this. "Sam?" I said, slipping out of bed. He was clicking away. "We can go." I stuck my head around the door frame.

"Are you sure?"

"Yes," I said.

The trail jutted downhill beside a wash, the grassland eroding at its edges into a fine orange-white dust. Spiky yucca replaced sage. The gold light deepened, late afternoon now, and when Sam stopped to let me catch up I couldn't help but catch his face in my hands. "You look so handsome in this light," I told him, but when I kissed him more insistently he pushed me away.

"Not here," he said.

The grassland from there betrayed white fins of rock, knee-deep canyons cut by flood, prickly pear crowning the tops of rises. We skipped deeper, pressing ourselves to flat, sun-warmed rocks or ducking into dark corners to see where they went. Simple clouds gathered in the sky. In the shadows the ground remained wet, the snow just melted earlier that day.

Somewhere just a few miles north of us, Wyoming began.

We took pictures of each other on the long flat path out of the badlands and toward the buttes, posing on giant chalky rocks. We leaned over to watch a giant anthill. When we approached the buttes Sam moaned, "I want to climb them!" and I laughed. They'd crumble in a second.

When the light dimmed, we walked back in the silver-gray grass, watching the sunset burn gold, then hot red, across the white windmills. By then we were quiet, our bodies in sync, climbing through the mud and dust. Our breaths warm and rhythmic. When we reached my Subaru he looked at me. "You okay to drive again?" and I said yes.

Later that night—after the final colors slipped from the sky, after we put on our favorite podcast and stopped in Greeley for burritos— he fell asleep in my passenger seat. And I didn't wake him as I drove through those dark farm towns. I didn't wake him, though my headache darkened and throbbed, because it was so sweet, the moonlight white across his cheekbone, the way his strong shoulders curled up inside his soft fleece. I didn't wake him because I was happy for him being there, because I loved him, even as my stomach twisted again, even as my eyes crossed with fatigue, as it got worse and worse. I didn't wake him. I loved him, and I would love him for a long time after, and I would never regret that last good day.

Not even with what happened to me after.

CAUSA FINALIS

CHAPTER 9

Boulder, Colorado
2010

ater, I would understand that to be sick is as much a way of seeing
the world as an acute condition. Once you have been seriously ill,
nothing is benign. A headache, a touch of nausea, a moment of
dizziness—these are not momentary conditions, resolved in a day or
fixed with a few ibuprofen, but the beginning of one's life vaulting in
some new and terrible direction. The body is not to be trusted.

To be well, then, is a sort of faith: a shrugging off of strange
sensations. A belief that the body is operating.

Which is why when you very badly want your body to be operating,
when you very badly want to believe you are well, you might grit
your teeth, dig your heels in, be emphatically *not sick*. Be *fine*. Ignore
the warning bells. To not be sick was to triumph over something, as
though the past year had been a choice I'd made that I could unmake
now, almost a year after I had passed out in that parking lot. As
though I could offer relief for everyone in my life by simply ignoring
the symptoms.

Which is why I left the house the next morning.

I'd woken up to a frantic text from my new supervisor, Danielle:
*Can you teach in Nederland today? Back is spasming so badly I can't
get up. I have a doctor's appointment at 10.* Lying in bed, holding the
phone, I was pleased she'd asked. It meant I'd earned her trust—

Nederland High School, located a half hour's drive up the winding cliffs of Boulder Canyon, was one of our best speaking engagements, with cheerful, curious students, a supportive teacher, and views of snow-encrusted peaks. Danielle had turned out to be one of the most dynamic people I'd ever met. As an employee, I wanted to impress her; as a human, I wanted to support her.

Of course, I texted back.

Then I stood up. My balance was all wrong. I staggered to the bathroom. The headache was back, and darker. Nausea knocked at me, and I swirled, clinging to the tile. How was I going to do this? I wanted desperately to call her back.

But I felt I couldn't. It was time not to be sick anymore. How hard could it be to stand up for an hour? I asked myself. For one hour, you can swallow this down. You can show up for Danielle.

How I came to be lying by the side of the road in Boulder Canyon is something of a blur. I had made it up into Nederland, gone through the roundabout, then gotten confused. There was no cell service. I couldn't think. I went into the visitors' center, thinking I might throw up. Every sensation so dense. My skin roiling. I made it back to my car and sat for a long time, moaning. *You have to get home.* The sloughing slopes of pine. The colorful miners' shacks. The road rose above the deep blue of the reservoir, the white concrete of the dam. I pulled over, wildly retching. The cliff there steep. The opposite bank full of houses made of glass. Nothing would come up. I lay there in the pine needles and gravel.

There was no sex ed, no Boulder, only my head, pressing in dark and terrible.

That voice again. *You have to get home.* Somehow driving the canyon. Sam's alarmed face when I burst through the door.

Then a week of this. It got better when I slept, but not for long. There was no eating. My fever was 102, then 102.7. I kept trying to show up to work—to the Teen Clinic, to the peer educator meeting at a nearby church—and despite my resolve I would become so dizzy and confused in the first blocks that I would turn around. "You look green," someone told me at the clinic when I made it all the way in, and I took home lists of primary care providers, calling everyone's doctors, trying to get in. Booked. No appointments for new patients. *It's got to be the flu,* I told myself each time I googled my symptoms. Each time I felt better after sleeping, I thought it would break. I didn't want more medical bills, I thought, flat against the bed.

Sam went to the nearby holistic pharmacy and talked to a naturopath. He brought home bottles of supplements. He refilled my water. But he was also supposed to leave that weekend on a ski expedition up Gannett Peak, in the Wind River Range, with a friend from Jackson. He was trying to get extra work done in advance of the trip, to stay out of freelancing trouble. Here I was again, needing his help. I could sense his brooding like a storm cloud, the sensation of being trapped.

By Friday morning a new feeling blossomed in me: one of terror. Something was very wrong. In Illinois, my parents were irate that I hadn't been to a doctor yet. Finally, I got an appointment with a practitioner near the hospital. "Why don't you walk?" Sam said darkly. "It's just five blocks." It was a workday. He had things to do. His friend had just bailed on him, so Sam was texting other climbing and skiing partners, trying to find somewhere else to spend the time off he'd banked. And there I was, pathetic and whimpering, breathing in gasps because my head hurt too much to inhale normally, shitting myself in small drips each time I took a step.

I asked again. He said no again.

I didn't want to make him. I thought about taking a cab. The logistics of a cab, the cost, in my brain, all fog. I couldn't think. It was so close.

"Please," I pleaded.

He took me.

I don't know how I made it down that long hallway at the doctor's office, bent over, so dizzy, shitting myself in public, *my head,* leaning onto a man who didn't want to be there. Sam filled out my paperwork while I lay as flat as I could in the waiting-room chair, the nausea surging, a violent wave.

Three months earlier, the business director at the clinic had pulled me aside. She was going to fudge the date of my hiring, she said, to make it a few weeks earlier. There was a three-month waiting period after hiring for insurance—and a six-month waiting period on preexisting conditions—which operated not in terms of actual dates but whole months. She knew I needed insurance as soon as possible. "Just in case someone asks," she said, winking at me, "you were hired February first."

Sam and I went to Pawnee Buttes on May 3. Which meant that, by the grace of the business director, I'd had functional insurance for three days.

Which was good, because the doctor sent me directly to the emergency room for a meningitis screening.

That day in the ER, the physician's assistant told me I had a gastrointestinal bug that had been going around. I fought him. "This started with a headache."

"Yeah." He puttered with my chart. "Everyone's been getting this."

"It's not gastrointestinal. That's not where it started."

"You'll just want to drink lots of water."

"I've drunk lots of water. The diarrhea didn't start until today, and I've been out the whole week." My voice was rising. "I was referred for meningitis. I need you to do a spinal tap and a CT. I'm not leaving until I receive the treatment I was referred for." When he pushed back, in my anger, I told him I wanted a *real* doctor, and the PA huffed out.

A physician took his place, one who spoke with the practiced gentleness that came with being handed one of those "difficult" patients. He ordered the CT and spinal tap.

The tests both came back negative. No meningitis, no brain tumor. But what? They discharged me without a diagnosis, handing me a prescription for Vicodin to help with the headache. "I'm scared," I told the doctor. "I don't see a route to getting better in what you're offering me. Something is wrong." There was nothing more they could offer me.

Terrified, I went back to bed. It was all I knew to do.

The next day, Sam received a call from an old friend coming through town. Knowing how disappointed he was about his trip, I encouraged him to meet her.

"You're really sick," he said.

"Yeah," I said. "And I'll still be sick when you get home. I'll probably just sleep. It's important that you get to take care of yourself, too."

In midafternoon, he headed off. I slept. And when I woke I watched the light dim from behind my headache, propping the laptop up on my legs, pushing in a DVD.

All at once the pictures in the movie started to become something wild and colorful and terrifying, shifting off the screen, becoming other things, and like a blossoming nightmare I thought I was supposed to do something with them, and a scream rose up in me and I slammed the computer shut and shoved it across the bed, because something had gone very, very wrong, the pain was rising up now, something had changed, something was very wrong in my brain, and I began calling Sam, calling and calling without answer. I called him again, called and texted, pictured him in the warm pub down on Pearl Street, laughing with his friend, on his second beer, the room loud and raucous, everyone's phones buried in their coats. Suddenly I knew that I might not make it if I waited for him. The hospital, four blocks away, was too far for me to walk at this point, too dangerous to drive now. And so I began calling everyone I knew who lived in Boulder, time becoming stretchy with panic. *Do I need an ambulance.*

PJ and Moss swept into the house, bundled me into the car. Our best clinic assistant and her husband. They took me back to the ER, shaking and pale, where PJ hassled everyone to move faster. "I'm going to put the IV in myself," she spat at one point, and I giggled. She actually could; it was part of her work during the clinic's abortion hours. "Nurse Ratched," she hissed at the nurse's retreating form, and gratitude filled me. Someone else was going to advocate for my care.

My blood cultures were still in the lab from the day before. The word came back: the samples were filled with bacteria. It was too soon to tell which.

Sam arrived just before I left the ER in a rolling bed, bound for the third floor.

The blur begins here. CT scans with contrast dye. Cold, lubricated ultrasound wands knobbing over my belly. Beating Heart Bear riding on my chest. A gallbladder full of pus. My spleen covered in blood clots. Someone told me they were going to take my gallbladder out, and Sam called my parents. My father on the phone from Illinois with the infectious disease doctor, with the gallbladder surgeon. Neither of them, he told me later, seemed to know of my heart history. My father calling Dr. Oza.

The flicker of a question: Had bacteria been implanted on my ICD?

Bacteremia is the presence of viable bacteria in the blood—what they call blood poisoning. The first symptoms are always chills, a sudden fever.

Sepsis is the whole-body inflammatory response to severe infection—a response that can cause multiple organ failure.

No-food-no-water-in-case-of-surgery-don't-tangle-the-IV-line-pushing-the-stand-to-the-bathroom-peeing-in-a-plastic-tray dark pain no breath.

My mother appeared.

In the hospital, work becomes a strange dream, clothing is impossible, the shopping center across the street a mirage. To walk to the bathroom is a million-mile journey. Money slips invisibly out of every fist, all these cups of pills, all these blood draws, all these jangling monitors.

I remember almost nothing: my mother bringing me all manner of food, feeding me delicate sips of Muscle Milk through a straw, trying to get me to eat. The oxygen line, burning my nostrils cold and raw, which sometimes fell out at night, the nurses racing in as my blood oxygen levels fell and the alarms shrieked. For three days, whenever I closed my eyes, bright, terrifying blasts of color formed shapes. Three men in chef's hats pushing a cast-iron pan full of breakfast toward me. A baby carriage in which the face of the baby was my own. My mother laughed when I told her about the images, writing them down in a small spiral notebook, but they felt toxic to me somehow, large and wild, like the place before death. She and Sam spirited fresh stacks of heated blankets into my room, rotating the thin blankets out as they cooled.

After a week of not being able to take a deep breath for the pain of the headache, I had pneumonia, my lungs gummy and impossible. I slept, nauseated, in fits. They took my blood pressure every three hours. The insides of my arms became black with the spreading bruises of IV tubing. Sam sat slumped in the corner with his laptop or was not there at all. His friends one night came with a casserole and paper bowls. Flowers arrived in a bright burst from the clinic.

In the cardiac cath lab, I gargled a numbing agent and swallowed a giant tube. They knocked me out to use it, to take pictures of my heart. They were trying to learn if I had a bacterial colony on my lead wire; they found a cluster of something but couldn't tell what. They would wait until I'd had more IV antibiotics, check again, see if it had changed. A lead wire with bacteria on it must come out, for bacteria make a refuge of foreign objects in the body, and the infection never goes away then, the heart inflaming and scarring dangerously. I didn't know then that this is sometimes how people end up on the transplant list.

On my fifth day in the hospital, my headache broke. My mother, after four days of stacking heated towels across my legs, peeled them off and helped me walk to the sink. There she carefully untied my smock and let it fall to the floor. For the first time, I looked up and saw my face in the mirror, gray and old looking. I brushed my teeth with my mother holding me steady, staring at myself. My belly was enormous, the organs inside it still inflamed, swollen with pus, and across it marched a long line of yellowing bruises where the nurses had jabbed in the day's heparin to keep the blood clots the body formed during sepsis from getting large enough to cause trouble. My chest was a graveyard of leftover adhesive, those neat brown edges where the EKG patches were placed, then ripped.

"I'm so sorry," I whispered, eyes filling with tears, putting down my toothbrush to cradle my stomach. "I'm so sorry."

In the shower I stood for a long time thinking about all the days I'd berated my body as fat, for not running fast enough, for being big-shouldered and big-hipped. For eye circles, for pimples, for wide feet and a big nose. For a heart defect. For having symptoms I didn't want. I understood, finally, that my body was real. It was not some illusion.

There was not some other version of it I would ever have. It was me, and I had almost lost it. We had almost been lost.

Now that I could walk, my mother and I took small loops through the hallway, pushing my IV stand. Walking required that I go off my oxygen for a few minutes, and I tired easily. Without the headache, I could finally cough out my pneumonia. I shuddered and hacked in long barks as we circled—until I pulled my weak chest muscles and the coughing began to send sharp pains across my front, down my arm.

On my last morning in the hospital, they wheeled me down to radiology to have a take-home IV line placed. Known as a PICC line—a peripherally inserted central catheter—the flexible tubing ran from the soft underside of my bicep up a vein to my heart. At home, I would inject my own antibiotics, which would be delivered to the house and stored in the refrigerator.

The tube unnerved me; more than a foot of it dangled out of my arm, with a little plastic bit on the end where I could control the flow, and a cotton wrap like the ribbed top of a sock to hold the plastic against my arm, where it couldn't get snagged on anything. A home nurse would come by to teach me in the morning, the tech told me. "You will not be able to shower unless you can wrap it very well in clear plastic wrap," she said. "You will need help. If you have a bathtub, that's best."

Goddamn bathtubless apartment, I thought for the millionth time.

Home nurse Sharon wore her hair in a tight bob and a smear of lipstick across her mouth. She showed up to the apartment early on our first morning together, a thing I was grateful for. I hadn't slept. My pulled chest muscles hurt so much I couldn't lie all the way down, and I kept making them worse with coughing. My first night home, I'd slept fitfully in the cushy pink chair, pulled up to the bed to lay my legs straight. Now I listened appreciatively as she showed me how to clear the line with saline, then use anticoagulant to keep it open, then clear it again with saline, then finally inject the antibiotic, Rocephin.

There was an art to this. You didn't want to inject it too fast.

The syringe stopper got a push every two minutes, a rush of icy-hot into my arm.

That night a friend of Sam's came up from Denver, plans they'd made a long time ago. We went for pizza. It felt good to sit in a booth, to be out in the world. But we'd walked, and on the way home the five blocks uphill proved too much, my skin turning sensitive again, the chills returning. It was still May, a wintry pinch to the mountain air after dark. Sam said he would go get the car, but we were halfway. It would be faster if I just kept going, I said, and made them wait for me. They were exasperated. At home, I collapsed. I'd taken on too much.

The next morning I woke with an enormous foot. All night I'd woken up in fits, coughing, my strained muscles sending razor slashes of pain across my body. I watched Sam sleep, calm beneath our red down covers. And then I tried to stand to go to the bathroom and found I had a clubfoot.

I touched it, the skin stretched and hard, not discolored, not painful, but weird-feeling. I limped to my laptop. The morning sun stretched through the windows. The late-season snow that had fallen while I was in the hospital had mostly shriveled into grass. Sam and I were supposed to visit our CSA farm for a meet and greet that afternoon. There would be a vegetable lunch, cheap local beer, and a chance to meet the other CSA members out on the East Boulder plains, under a white tent in the grass.

But I had to: I googled the foot. Again and again I read the same word, the one I'd been thinking: *embolism*. Blood clot. I waited for Sharon.

It happened as though in a dream: the quick knock, Sharon's cheery face, Sam stumbling past us in his boxers to use the restroom, Sharon's face falling as she looked at my foot. She took my temperature, my blood pressure, my respiration rates and pulse. I told her the shooting pains across my chest were just as bad as they had been, so bad I couldn't laugh, couldn't sleep, could barely take a deep breath. She held my left foot in her hands, her blue eyes sorrowful. In the next room, Sam was preparing for our picnic: putting his jeans on, choosing a T-shirt. In this room, we were talking about the way blood clots could dislodge, careening toward important body parts, cutting off blood supply to the brain or lungs.

"You have to go in," she said. "They might clear you right away. But the risk is too high. You have to go in."

This time I packed a small bag with sweatpants, toothbrush, and bears because I understood that sometimes you go into the hospital and you just don't come out. I could still picture us at the farm, laughing about the bag in the car and how unnecessary it was, because I was young, because I was healthy. And yet when the ER doctor reviewed my chart he got a very serious look on his face.

By then breathing hurt so much I wanted to scream. I took air in slivers, knowing that it wasn't good for my pneumonia. Sam looked past me, lost, slumped in the same gray visitor's chair. We were silent. Then, out of nowhere, he said, "This fucking sucks."

"Yes," I said quietly, "it does."

When the nurse asked me what I wanted, I almost yelled. "Morphine." And I got morphine, a bright push of it sliding through me, clearing the static from my mind, filling my limbs with a warm peace. *So that's why people do heroin,* I thought. Then they took me back to the third floor.

"Your legs are clear," a doctor told me upstairs. "But we can't rule out a clot."

"I'm supposed to be on a farm," I said.

My new room was around the corner from my old room. This time the window overlooked roof tiles covered in gravel, great whirring fans. Something in me was changing, shifting and hardening. In the small square out my window, a young aspen stretched thinly upward. I couldn't imagine why it was on the roof of the hospital. But like a plant to a prisoner, it became the only thing I could look at.

"You could go without me," I turned to Sam.

He scoffed. "I'm not going without you," he said.

He went down to the parking lot to call my parents. In the meantime, an aide swept me away for another CT with contrast—the dye that makes you feel like you're peeing your pants. When they pushed it into my IV, it flooded me with such a burning, nauseating warmth I wanted to die.

Then X-rays. Because of my painful chest the aides gripped my hands, lowering me down to where the machines needed me, as I gasped and cried out.

When I arrived back in my room, a nurse from the previous week ducked her head in. "Oh, no," she said. "I didn't want to be seeing you."

"I know," I said.

"I saw your name on the chart, and my heart sank," she said. When she told me they were keeping me overnight, though, I was almost relieved: for the angled bed, for the morphine. The most terrible truth was that I knew I needed to be there. I needed the world designed for the sick, manned by capable people willing to care for me. I couldn't take care of myself—and Sam couldn't take care of me either.

The next morning, as the aide was rolling me past the nurses' station, I saw a tall man out of the corner of my eye and did a double take. "Dad!" I said.

My father's face split open to see me. Though he was smiling, he was also, I knew, taking in the hospital gown, the IV bag, the puffiness in my face. I was returning from another round of the numbing gargle, the plastic tube down the throat, Dr. Oza taking pictures of my heart, and I was woozy, my throat sore.

He looked sheepish. "I got scared," he said.

In my room, he told me he'd noticed an article in the *Chicago Tribune* about hospital infection rates. "It got me wondering," he said, and he told me he'd looked up Boulder Community Hospital's rates online. What he found did not soothe him, and he went down a rabbit hole, reading about sepsis and the way the body's immune response to infection could generate so many tiny blood clots that they could begin to reduce blood flow, cutting off organs. "I got freaked out," he said, and it became worse when Sam called to let them know the doctors suspected a clot, which—dislodged from the leg—could clog the lungs, causing tissue death, or go to the brain, causing aneurysm and stroke. "I'm going out there," he told my mother. "I just need to eyeball her. I need to talk to the doctors myself and assess the situation." He bought himself a ticket. Here he was.

He pulled a book out of his bag, a copy of Shel Silverstein's *A Light in the Attic,* which he'd bought me when I was a kid. "I thought we could read together," he said, sheepish again, and my heart broke as I saw how much he feared he might lose me.

Not long after, they found the pulmonary embolism. One of the hospitalists showed me the X-ray, the gray cluster in my lung. The pneumonia made it hard to tell what was what. Was it related to my foot? No one could say, but my foot had deflated and I was back to just chest pain, like a dagger slashing skin.

In midafternoon, a pharmacist appeared in the doorway and began explaining a new drug. A stack of papers fluttered in her hand.

"Wait, what?" I said.

She looked uncomfortable. "Coumadin," she said. "It's a more powerful anticoagulant than the heparin shots you've been getting in your belly. The hospitalists prescribed it to break up the clot in your lung. To prevent more."

No one said anything, so she continued.

"You'll need to come back to the hospital weekly," she said, "for six months."

My breath caught. "Six months?"

"You'll need to avoid vitamin K—you know, leafy greens. It's the antidote to this medication—it causes it not to work. Kale is a big problem."

"It's farmer's market season," I said.

The pharmacist smiled tightly, shifted. "Well, it's not that you can't have any," she said. "You just have to have the same amount every week so your dosage works. You have to be really careful." She lifted a few papers. "I have some handouts for you if you want them. You'll have to watch your activity level. Coumadin induces hemophilia. You'll want to avoid activities where you might fall down or get scratched. A wound may keep bleeding because of the blood thinner."

"And what if I don't want this?" I said. Panic was welling up, metallic in my mouth, and I wished I could breathe deeply.

"Well, it's been prescribed," she said lamely. "The hospitalists have determined that it's essential to your safety." I was working to control myself when she said, "You've already had your first dose."

"What?"

"A nurse administered—"

"Without telling me what it *was*?" I said. The tears were coming hard and fast. Rage. Then I remembered. The nurse who, earlier, had come around the side of the bed and jabbed me in the stomach with a needle, the way they did when they administered heparin. Except this woman had said nothing—no hello, no warning. It must have been a different drug.

"It's medically necessary," the pharmacist said again.

"Out," I said. I could barely get the words out, I was crying so hard, each gulp rippling across my chest like a hot poker.

"Kati," my dad said.

"I—am—twenty—four—years—old," I gasped. "And I am not going to the hospital every fucking week—"

"Do you need some—"

"OUT!" I said. "Everybody out."

In the quiet after the door clicked shut, I watched the aspen, blurred by tears, shift in the breeze, in its sorry little pen. Every part of me felt hot and sharp. I was just then hitting the six-month mark on my lead wire. The greatest risk, I'd thought, had passed. I'd imagined I could begin my return to things; I could stop living in fear.

But if I were on Coumadin, I'd have to start over. Six months as a hemophiliac, worrying about falling or getting scratched. I wouldn't be free of this place, even after I left.

I knew then that I would die young. Something had collapsed in me those weeks, a belief in the privilege youth had once afforded—this sense that I could carry on living and generally be left alone. I had almost rotted alive for reasons no one seemed to understand. I had gone into cardiac arrest in a parking lot. I'd had microelectronics implanted in my body solely to make death go away, but there it was still, and there it would always be. It had always been there; I just hadn't seen it. The ICD seemed now grotesque, an absurd idea.

All that effort, only to rot in the ground anyway.

Out the window, dark clouds churned over Mount Sanitas, one of those big spring storms that sweep down the Front Range and out over the plains. After the rain would come sun, and after the sun would come kale, and I wanted to be browsing the farmer's market, shoving greens into my mouth, then going for raucous runs on the mountainside. I wanted it, even if it meant I would die. It was, I realized now, what it meant to be alive.

Eventually my father stuck his head back through the door. "Can I come in?" he asked, his voice tender, and I nodded. My breathing was stilled. He opened the door, and Sam followed him inside, looking overwhelmed.

"Dad," I said, "will you read Shel Silverstein to me?"

"Of course," he said, pulling out the white volume he had brought, flipping to our old favorite poems. The sound of his voice made me want to cry out of sweetness, but instead I settled back into it. I took careful, measured breaths into the deepest part of my lungs.

Later, we ordered Thai from the little restaurant next to the University Inn, pulling the chairs around the nightstand we used as our table. There, my dad pulled out a DVD: Ken Burns's documentary on the Dust Bowl. "No one else would watch it with me," he announced. "I thought you'd think it was cool." Even though it hurt my chest, I laughed hard. The nightstand became our laptop stand, the two men pulled their chairs close to my bed, and we watched as the clouds took over.

What my body knew my infectious disease doctor confirmed: I likely didn't need the Coumadin. Dr. Todd Turner—tall, slouchy, and awkwardly endearing—listened carefully as I told him what had happened. "I'm not sure that's appropriate," he said, leaning back against the wall. "Coumadin is a strong drug. It's also used commercially as a rat poison." He shrugged. "It's a blood thinner. It makes them bleed out."

"The conversation, in your case," he told me, "is *what* exactly is in the bottom of your left lung. We can't exactly see, because of your pneumonia." He explained to me that some blood clots form naturally in the body as part of the healing mechanism—like the clots that close wounds. These are called thrombuses, and it would make sense to have one in my lungs because of the pneumonia.

But if the clot in my lung had come from my leg—if it had stopped blood at my foot before migrating farther into the body—that was problematic. The question was whether I would generate more clots. "Your age is a major consideration," he said. "Many older adults start having repeat embolisms, and Coumadin would be a good cautionary measure. But that's unlikely to be true for you. You're at higher risk from being stationary in the hospital, but that's why they've been giving you Fragmin or heparin shots every day."

"Can you get them to take me off it?" I said.

He smiled. "I want to hear the hospitalists' rationale, but I suspect they're just being overly cautious. I'll come back in a bit and tell you what I find."

The morning of my discharge, my dad pulled his big black rental SUV up to the entrance while an aide wheeled me down. Rain smacked the windshield as soon as I was in. I cracked the window. Everything smelled fresh and alive, the wet blacktop, the living grass. I was drunk on non-recycled air, on color and sound. We ate lunch downtown at a panini shop, a block-long walk that left me pausing for breath against a tree, my IV line snug against my arm. I felt old, like I'd been plucked out of this world years ago, and I wondered if I would ever fit inside it again.

Yet something in me felt strangely strong and clear. The part of me that had grown blurry and unmoored over the long year since I'd passed out suddenly snapped into focus.

On the third night after my discharge, Sam told me he wanted to cook a welcome home dinner. But he seemed angry as he cooked it, his hair growing tall from how he grabbed it in stress. He had outbursts at the tomatoes, muttered at the chicken. By the time he set the meal on the table, I wasn't sure it was for welcoming me.

"Do you like me?" I found myself saying suddenly. He froze. What I would and wouldn't take from him had changed. "Do you think I'm pretty? Are you attracted to me? Do you think I'm funny? Do you want to spend time with me?"

And he put down his fork, his face full of answers.

"I always assumed the problem was these things that kept happening to us," he said. "But what if it's *us*? What if it never stops?"

For weeks, then, fighting. Though he'd been working from the house for the better part of a year, he had a desk half an hour away that a nonprofit had offered to let him use, which he rarely did. That week he began slipping out early each morning to drive there, leaving me alone in the house to do my injections, to wrestle a roll of Saran wrap with my nondominant hand, trying to wrap my PICC line tightly enough so I could shower. Too often, I failed, driving to work with greasy hair plastered to my forehead. Our fridge was full of rotten food and boxes of antibiotic, heparin, and saline.

I practiced walking down the block. I had become so very weak. But now I was awake, and I saw him. Anger ran hot in me.

I had begun calling him my partner and not my boyfriend when he moved to Boulder, but he did not feel like my partner now.

One night, in the middle of a spat, he turned to me helplessly. "Honestly, Kati?" he said. "I don't think this is going to work out."

"Fine," I said, but the tears were erupting. I slipped out the front door, sat quietly on the stoop with my head in my hands. Finally, I went to get my purse. "I'm going downtown," I told Sam, voice quavering, sliding by him.

He stopped me, placed his bearded cheek against mine the way we always had. I could feel his grief.

I went wordlessly out of the house.

At the wine bar, on the same patio where I had once called my parents to tell them Dr. Oza thought I needed a defibrillator, the same patio where my mom had told me I would need to live in Boulder for more than six months, I ordered the sweetest white they had. *What you drink at the end to make the bitter taste better*, I texted my mom. I stayed as late as I could.

Sam waited up, worried about me. "Have you eaten?" he said when at last I let myself into the house.

"No," I said. "Just lots of dessert wine." And he took out the leftovers from the Indian food he had ordered, and he brought them to me in bed, and he sat beside me as I ate them, the room full of our sadness.

For a week I woke up sobbing in the middle of the night, and he held me. Then on the morning before my twenty-fifth birthday, he came to me and said, "I think I need to go to the Cape for the summer."

"Okay," I said, looking into his sad eyes. It felt at first like a temporary separation, a way to get breathing room; he could stay at his uncle's place for free and keep paying rent on our apartment. But within days he'd decided not to leave his things, and I came home from the clinic one Saturday night to find the house torn apart— the spice rack pulled off the wall and dismantled, his books removed from my shelves, papers stacked in the middle of the room. The grief that filled me then was so large that I walked back down to my car and returned to the clinic, punching in the code to let myself into the dark building, working alone upstairs until almost midnight to put off confronting what had become of things.

We fought less once we'd broken up. It was good for us, like a patient whose terminal diagnosis allows him to finally set the right priorities. Now the end was in sight. We woke each other to fevered, wordless sex in the middle of the night and met for lunch by the river, eating burritos and kissing in the downed cottonwood leaves. During those weeks a sudden heat descended, and up on the Divide the big mountains began sweating hard into the reservoirs. Downtown, the creek had jumped its banks, closing the underpasses and pushing into the trees. I wanted to be in that current, lifted off my feet, carried downstream in the hand of violence, past the grief of the separation that was coming. Bumping up over the rocks. The mountains hazy and blue with heat.

On the day Sam left for the Cape, I told Danielle I would be in late. Sam and I woke in each other's arms knowing this was it—after all the months of fighting and weeks of crying. It was June twenty-fifth, our two-year anniversary. It had been one year and one week since I passed out in the parking lot in Jackson.

We had the sex of people who know each other's bodies by heart, only now there was some other depth layered onto it. Like a poem, memorized, the familiar coming-around of sound; the way, on a mountain highway, one anticipates the most beautiful curves, and yet the colors still hold something new. Love was not our problem, I knew, clasping his head in my hands, feeling the strength of his thighs—but all that had happened to us seemed too close and too complicated to know yet what was.

When we were done, I felt anxiety twist in me. "I should go to work," I said.

His face looked frantic. "You said we could go have crepes for breakfast!"

He was right. I had. But I wanted to slip out, to slip away, to use my responsibilities to cut this short, to avoid the unbearable grief. I also knew I wouldn't be able to live with myself if I didn't have this last morning with him.

We showered, dressed, walked the five blocks to the crepe shop where we sometimes worked together the previous winter, side by side on our laptops, each of us getting a savory crepe and then sharing a sweet one, drinking coffee or sangria as the front window fogged against the cold. Now it was June, and the heat was here. We held hands. We sat at an outdoor table against the loud street, and we talked about his trip. How far he would drive each day. What I should do with our CSA share. How we would pay for the storage unit we had shared since our move, which now held all his belongings. It was a shared life until the moment we cleaved it. He looked beautiful in that light. It was impossible that he was leaving.

But then we walked up the hill to the house, and there was nothing left to do. In the doorway, I cried and cried.

"Lady," he said, holding me. He pressed his bearded cheek to mine.

"Text me when you go," I told him, "so I know for sure. So we don't have to do this again."

He came through the doorway with me, watched me sobbing into my hands. "I just want to take it from you," he cried out, "so you can be happy." I nodded. He closed the door.

Then he opened it, peeked out at me. He stood on the steps and watched me go down.

The last thing I saw of him that day on Maxwell Avenue was his face in the bedroom window, holding up Beary's paw, both of them waving goodbye.

I would never know why I went septic. My dad remains convinced the bacteria were implanted with my defibrillator, as is a distinct risk with that surgery. Ever skeptical of the medical industry, he wondered if the hospital wanted to avoid a lawsuit for implantation of bacteria, if this shirking of liability was the real reason the dots didn't get connected.

That the device remained inside me, though, is the most solid evidence I have that this is not true. The device remained inside me for the full span of its life, and no infection ever returned.

Group B streptococcus does not often turn to sepsis. It lives benignly in our digestive tracts, in our anuses and vaginas. When the bacteria enter the bloodstream and suddenly proliferate, triggering the inflammation of sepsis, it is most often in babies sliding through the birth canal, or in new mothers, ripped up by birth, or in the elderly and immunosuppressed, whose defenses are tired.

It turns out that what lives inside us has always been capable of causing our deaths, if we get too tired to push back. It turns out that life requires a subtle, constant pushing. A sweet work that some of us can no longer show up for.

It might have been a surprise to others that I was vulnerable to what lived inside me, that I was so very tired. There are those who sing the gospel of the resilience of the young. But it was not surprising to me. That spring I had gone downstairs at work to be swabbed by the clinic nurses more times than I cared to admit, with enormous overgrowths of bacterial vaginitis that kept me up at night itching. That I would lack the basic resources to fight off Group B strep at the end of that very long year, when my body was trying to heal not just a wound but a way of life that had shattered—a spring in which I worked every hour I could to pay a mountain of medical bills—a spring in which I fought with the man I loved, in which I felt our relationship made conditional by health, in which I had begun swallowing shards of betrayal, absorbing the ways he failed me at the moments that mattered most—

I find it unsurprising that this could kill a person.

In my body lived death. It had always been there. Perhaps it was sex itself, the love of Sam at the end of all this, that cut an entrance into my blood: some tiny final ripping sound no one would ever hear, something a woman less beaten could have healed.

But I wasn't that woman anymore.

CAUSA FORMALIS

CHAPTER 10

Tucson, Arizona
2012

On the night of the shocks, a lone police officer arrived first, a dark shadow coming across the field from where he'd left his cruiser on the street. "Someone here call 911?" he said, his eyes finding me on the ground, where I lay in the center of the crowd. The ambulance, he reported, was lost. He made sure I was stable, then awkwardly stepped aside to send directions.

Someone tucked a sweatshirt over me. One of my teammates rubbed my arm. "Do you need us to call someone?" people kept asking.

"Not yet," I said, thinking of Christine, so far away. Stalling on the moment my parents would receive this phone call.

From my spot on the ground beneath the bright lights, one star was visible. I could smell only my own burned tissues.

The paramedics drove the ambulance onto the soccer field and tumbled out. Their faces appeared above me, illuminated by stadium lights, blue-eyed and concerned, and things sped up. Did I know who I was? Did I know where I was? Thick fireman hands slid a blood pressure cuff over my bicep, carefully lifted my shirt to affix electrodes. As one man at a time began asking me technical questions—*How long have you had the device? What condition is it for? Do you take any medications?*—I had the slow sensation of coming back into a story I'd forgotten was mine. I had been an expatriate, living among the well. These men recognized me for what I was, and I responded in their language.

It is hard to pinpoint when, after sepsis, I'd crossed the border into safety. All that first summer, I lived with the terror of one whose body could go off the rails at any moment. Every headache was sepsis's return. I went to the hospital early one morning when I was due at a work conference after a series of chest pains had me convinced the blood clot was still lurking in my lung, that I'd been wrong to refuse the Coumadin. It had been less than two months since my last discharge. The emergency room doctor looked at me gravely as he read my chart, informing me that although I'd received too much radiation as a young person, because of my medical history it was worth running another scan to make sure the clot was gone. I had packed a bag, had brought the bears. I was keenly aware that this time I was alone.

But the scan was clear; the clot was gone. The pain must have been muscular, a pulled pectoral. I arrived at the conference, slipping quietly into the empty seat beside Danielle as a speaker flicked through a PowerPoint. I spread pats of butter on my roll, forked at the lettuce on my plate, and opened my shiny folder. Danielle and I kept looking at each other.

"I can't believe you are here," she whispered.

"I can't believe I am, either."

And so the privilege of my youth returned; my body became gloriously silent. My follow-up appointments were unremarkable. During the quiet evenings I now spent alone, I ran the ridgelines of the mountain I had looked at so longingly from the inside of the hospital. I ran hard, gulping air. Leaping rock to rock. Outpacing the ghosts beneath the pines.

Slowly, then quickly, my body regained its strength. On lunch breaks I walked two doors down to the climbing gym with the clinic assistants to boulder—first cautiously, and then with the familiarity of one who has been climbing all her life. Christine and I began to coordinate our device checks at Dr. Oza's office, sometimes walking the half mile together from my apartment, sitting together in that waiting room at the end of my street: still the only two young patients. The St. Jude technician would motion us back at the same time, and in the small room where the device carts sat, one after the other we would have the wand draped over our devices, watching each other grimace as the tech raced and slowed our hearts.

Eventually, even the lingering hospital bills were gone. In August—two months after I finally had my PICC line removed—my parents came to Colorado to visit Rocky Mountain National Park. We all noted: it was a trip to Colorado that did not involve a hospital! All summer I'd relied on Sam's rent checks crossing the country to me in small envelopes, covering half the cost of our little apartment on Maxwell. But soon he'd be returning and renting his own place, and I'd be on my own. I couldn't afford it. At the time, I was still making payments to medical offices across town, for both the out-of-pocket implantation and my copays after sepsis. During the long weeks of sepsis, I'd lost my second job helping write that corporate water conservation book, and I knew I couldn't work a second job anyway. I felt inside me a new sort of gauge for what was sustainable and what wasn't, having learned the lesson that the way I lived could kill me, that small stresses added up in the body. Though I met with a few potential roommates, I knew in my heart that moving in with others somewhere else would be too much for me, and I resisted the idea of adding a long commute from a cheaper part of the Front Range to my already long days driving between schools all over the county. More important, the thought of leaving the apartment, my refuge over a year of tumult, filled me with sorrow. The sunlight filtering through maple leaves, the gleaming wood floors, the quiet walk to Mount Sanitas, my composter out back just beginning to make fertile what had rotted during sepsis—all this steadied me. And I craved steadiness with a desperation I almost couldn't bear to admit.

One afternoon, my dad took me for a walk up and down the hilly blocks of Mapleton Hill. "I've been thinking," he told me. "You didn't choose all this. The debt you're carrying because of what happened with your heart and sepsis. You're so young." He had inherited an account when his father died three years previously, he told me, and he was required to take a certain amount of money out of it every year. He admired my attempts to be financially independent again, he said, but he wanted to use this money to help make my payments.

I cried at his kindness. I knew that the chances I was receiving to start fresh were rare and privileged, and that they would change the course of my life.

Over the following six months he would clear more than $6,000 off my plate. Eventually, to earn extra money to pay for my ongoing health-care costs, I began renting my house out online and camping, or sleeping in my car for a few nights at a time on Boulder's leafy streets. I would stay in my sun-dappled apartment in the trees until I left Boulder for good.

The ICD became a story, then: the reason I'd moved to Boulder; the reason for neck and back pain I could never quite shake after the immobilization of my left side; the reason I bought only that one sports bra with the angled strap, and always two sizes too small. The longer the ICD remained silent, the less I thought about it in a serious way, in a fearful way. Time after time when I thought the device should have recorded something, nothing was there.

Once there were men, the scar that rested over my left breast became a test of sorts, a measurement of whether they could stand to hear about the death that was in me, whether they knew how to respond to suffering or became awkward, even nauseated, when told what the scar was from.

I knew how to be fun with them, cheerful and flippant. But I wasn't stupid.

I told myself: for the rest of your life you will have heart surgeries. You must keep in your life only men who will be good in the hospital.

The Affordable Care Act, known more widely as Obamacare, passed in March of 2010. The law would theoretically make it possible for me to purchase my own private health insurance on a federal marketplace, barring insurers from discriminating against my "preexisting condition." But in 2011, when I began applying to graduate school, the details still felt foggy. As I hunched over my laptop at late-night coffee shops on the Pearl Street Mall, drafting and redrafting my application materials, the law hung in the balance, the subject of a suit by twenty-eight Republican state attorneys general who were hoping to have it overturned as unconstitutional. Working in academia, I hoped, would give me a buffer against the political winds as I surrendered my insurance from the health clinic.

In the beginning, I planned to apply to eight master of fine arts creative writing programs all over the country. In the end, land tugged at me: I didn't want to leave the interior West, its big empty spaces and fierce sun. In the spring of 2012, I put in notice at work: I would leave on July 3, a date chosen to secure health insurance for the month. On August 1, I would move to Tucson, to enroll at the University of Arizona.

Now, on the soccer field, the paramedics eased up my shirt to place adhesive electrodes on my ribs and sternum. The first EKG came back normal—no sign of the torsades de pointes rhythm—and one of the paramedics gently asked, "Do you think you can sit up?" I nodded. An EMT supported me from behind, watching my heartbeat. Then standing: still good.

"How do you feel?" one of the paramedics said. "Any different standing? Are you dizzy at all?" The question hung in the air. They were asking the same question I was asking myself: Had my life just been saved or not? Why had the device gone off if I never lost consciousness? And if it was malfunctioning, why had it stopped shocking me?

"Honestly," another said, looking at me seriously, "with no arrhythmia present on the EKG, if you don't think you had a syncope tonight, all the emergency room can do is waste your money."

"That's what I was thinking," I said. I'd been to enough emergency departments, they could tell, to play this one to the end: a long wait, surrounded by coughing kids and bleary-looking adults; a conversation about how I'd gotten a referral from Campus Health for cardiology but hadn't been in yet; being told my heart enzymes were normal. At best, they'd interrogate my device—which would be cheaper in the pacemaker clinic than in the emergency room, with its required copay—and maybe send me on for an X-ray if they suspected my wire had moved like Christine's. Taking two thousand volts to the heart felt like an emergency, but it wasn't one.

"As long as it has stopped shocking you," the EMT added. "If it starts shocking you again or you have symptoms, go in. Call your cardiology office—someone will be on call and you can see if they tell you the same thing. Probably they'll just want to see you first thing in the morning."

Then he tilted his head at me. "If you need to turn it off in an emergency, to make it stop, put a magnet over it."

Then the paramedics were packing up, and everyone who stood around me began to shake out of their daze. The game was over. It had been a forfeit anyway—not enough female players on one of the teams. No one had any interest in trying to start up again. As the players drifted back to where their jackets and water bottles waited on the sidelines, I turned to my friend Julien, whom I'd come with. His eyes were red. Whatever strength had come over me, taking deep breaths as two thousand volts rolled into my heart, answering technical questions for the EMTs—it all evaporated. I collapsed into his shirt. Weak. Shaking with tears.

I remembered the afternoon he asked me to join the team. We were walking back to my house after class, on a street gritty with gravel and potholes, the afternoon light turning that shade of gold the desert is known for. Julien—the man I'd been referring to as my gay husband since our first day of grad school, when we platonically fell into one of those wonderful, immediate friendships—had been agitating within the English department, trying to pull together the number of players we needed. On that day, as I pushed my bike beside him, I considered my response.

"I'm not supposed to," I admitted. "I mean I'm not *allowed* to, officially. No contact sports."

But I had played soccer from fourth grade until junior year of high school, often the MVP, several times as the captain, and in college I'd gained the nickname Tank for the way I barreled into a crowd of players and emerged with the ball. I missed that kind of running, the deftness of a fake, the pleasure of a crisp pass. I knew that taking a ball or an elbow to the chest could be problematic for the device, and I'd been told that sprinting was the worst form of exercise for an LQT type 2, but it was hard to view soccer as dangerous. It had been three years since the ICD's implantation, and nothing had happened. I'd run hard up mountains. I'd startled in the middle of the night in Sierra Leone when a man rattled our windows trying to break in, my heart nearly beating out of my chest. I'd sobbed hysterically after a man I'd been seeing glumly refused to kiss me. In all these instances, nothing had shown up at my device check. Instead, the technicians asked me questions like: "Um, did you pass a giant magnet at 9:51 p.m. on August twenty-second? The polarity of your heartbeat reversed. I mean, it was fine. It's just really weird." (In that instance, we spent a few minutes brainstorming about armored trucks and magnetic necklaces and bracelets before we figured out I'd been on a bad date and had held up my bike saddlebags—which had magnetic handles—in front of my chest to prevent an unwanted lean-in.)

If I'd been able to ski and climb and run without jostling the wire in my chest—if every workout and honked horn and loud alarm that made me nervous had so far been fine—what, exactly, was the risk? What would trigger this long QT type 2 adrenaline-startle response thing I'd lived so in terror of?

When I asked my body whether or not I should join the intramural soccer team, maneuvering my bike around the potholes, I was surprised to hear it telling me two things simultaneously: that I should say yes. And that something would happen.

"I'm just your sub," I told Julien fiercely, jabbing my finger at him. "I get to decide how much I play and when."

"Of course," he said, but he was laughing, so pleased.

There was, of course, one more factor at play. The other thing my body told me to do that fall was to go off beta-blockers.

After three years on the medication, my heart was still maxing out at 130 beats per minute. That had been enough to return to activity, but it meant never quite being able to push myself the way I wanted. My ability to have a sex life had improved, but I still lived with a strange throat-constricting sensation, and I could barely operate at the high altitudes I used to love.

I had begun to think about type 2 long QT in theoreticals. If the arrhythmia had to do with adrenaline spikes in the body, would strengthening the ability of my nervous system to downregulate itself after those spikes be helpful? I could not control a honking horn, but I could to some extent manage the emotional side of the trigger. If my body managed its stress well, how carved in stone was it that my QT interval would lengthen? And if it did, by how much would it lengthen? Would the arrhythmia, if it formed, just cause a few weird beats, or would it necessarily spiral out of control into cardiac arrest?

I got the sense, from researching, that we simply didn't know yet.

The spring before I moved to Arizona, I had committed to deep and painful bodywork with a massage therapist who seemed to know where every bit of the trauma of my sick year was hiding out in my body. At his suggestion, I had committed to a weekly yoga practice. I began meditating. I received weekly acupuncture. All these are known to strengthen the parasympathetic nervous system, decreasing one's reactivity. I knew, though, that my job at the clinic was still too stressful for me to transition off the beta-blockers; in my final six months there, Danielle had abruptly left for a new job, following her partner to Salt Lake City, and I'd had to keep both our jobs afloat—working long and erratic hours—while the clinic hired a replacement. It wasn't until I got to Tucson, starting a new life that seemed to suit me so much better, that I felt like it was time. Graduate school was a lot of work, but it was largely work I scheduled myself, spending long days on a single task, never missing yoga or trail running because of work. Classes unfolded predictably, clumped on two or three days of the week, and instead of driving across a metropolitan area in a blizzard during rush hour, as I had in Colorado, I simply hopped on my bike and coasted the mile to campus, the weather always clear, if hot. I'd moved into a little 1930s adobe house with a palm tree out front and palo verde, mesquite, and salt cedar trees casting shade into the yard. The inside of the house held a graceful sort of calm, the tile an orange saltillo, desert light pouring through the windows.

I knew you couldn't just stop taking beta-blockers; you had to slowly transition yourself off. I knew, also, that no doctor would be willing to work with me on this. And so I told a few friends—enough so that if something did happen there would be no mystery—and I called my sister.

"I understand," she said. "You have to know. I already know, for myself." She'd had torsades de pointes even *on* beta-blockers. "But your case is different."

She was saying it in terms I had overlooked, at least consciously. This was about whether I needed the beta-blockers, of course. But it was also about the ICD itself. I was grasping for some kind of reassurance, some kind of indication of the ground I stood on. Without the drugs, would I be passing out all the time, taking shocks over and over? Could the defibrillator be a quiet backup in a beta-blocker-free life?

Might it even be an unnecessary appendage?

There are those who say our genes are our gods. I chose not to listen. I backed my dose down over the course of three weeks. By October, I was quietly beta-blocker free.

We walked to Julien's car in the dark, my Thermos of tea still warm in my hand, each step feeling tentative. Julien would drive me to get a milkshake—the only thing open so late on a Sunday night was the Baskin-Robbins on Speedway—where I found myself almost embarrassed to want so badly this particular type of comfort. Soupy vanilla, small black chips of chocolate. Back at my house, he sat on my cheap black couch while I called my parents.

It was a call that felt like two calls: not only that I had been shocked but also that I was off beta-blockers. That I was unsure the role this had played in the evening. My parents were calmer than I had anticipated; but then, they'd gotten good at these calls—these dramatic turns of events, their daughters thousands of miles away. Whatever reservations they had or judgments they were making would usually come later.

Although my mother couldn't resist saying, "You shouldn't have been playing soccer anyway."

I caught Christine in bed, reading in a pile of pillows. "Three times in a row," she kept saying. "Three times in a row!" Unlike everyone else, she could actually imagine what this felt like. I pictured her in a tank top, blond hair falling over her shoulders, touching the pale earthworm scar above her left breast. By then she was twenty-four years old, the age I'd been when I first passed out, and she wept and wept, her voice growing clotted with snot and emotion. I was again forcing her to confront something she had moved on from as quickly as possible. Her first shock when the wire moved inside her heart. Her second shock while running. Her third shock in a lap pool during a lifeguard competition, after she won an event that required retrieving a dummy from the pool floor. The fourth shock—one morning in bed when her alarm went off—which had saved her life. When I told her I thought I had smelled burning, she said wryly, "I always assumed my tissues were cooked."

She told me she didn't think she would sleep that night. "I'm suddenly terrified it's going to go off. I know that's crazy. But I'd forgotten about it, and now I remember again."

"It's so awful," I said.

"Yes," she said. "Now you know what I meant."

"Why this time?" she asked, and kept asking. And then I cried again, too, for the way she had gone right to it, the most important question, the question we needed an answer for, in order to know how to live. "I can't believe I went to the amusement park," she told me. "I can't believe I went to the haunted house. I can't believe I forgot."

Sometime before midnight, Julien went home. I took a leftover beta-blocker from the bottle I kept in my nightstand, and I put myself to bed, fighting my fear of being alone with the reasoning that I'd had no actual cardiac symptoms all evening.

The next morning, I woke early and called the hospital. The pacemaker clinic could fit me in. I drove myself; somehow the risk of being shocked while driving seemed more tenable than while biking, although in every way I felt tender, uncertain about my safety.

In the narrow clinic, crowded with interrogation machines specific to the various heart-rhythm device manufacturers, the tech draped the St. Jude Medical wand over my ICD and clicked at the computer, barely looking at me. Although he knew I'd come in because I'd taken three shocks to the heart, he did not ask how I was. When I told him I no longer took my medication, he rolled his eyes, shook his head. "Take your medication," he said. "Or stop working out. Simple."

"Doesn't look like you had an arrhythmia," he said after a few minutes. "Doesn't look like there's anything wrong with the device, either. The settings are just too low." He chuckled.

"These would be good settings for a fifty-five- or sixty-year old." This did not surprise me, knowing how fiercely protective Dr. Oza had been, how afraid in the early years. And yet a bright surge of anger flooded my chest, for the continual insult of receiving care meant for someone nearer to the end than the beginning of their life.

When the electrophysiologist came in—a quiet, mousy-looking blond woman with glasses whom I hadn't met yet—she pushed the buttons to change my settings, increasing my threshold to above 210 beats per minute, a rate it was unlikely I'd hit during exercise, with or without beta-blockers. But when she finished, she never turned to me. She did not ask me how I was. She did not ask my reasoning for going off beta-blockers. She simply picked up her prescription pad, wrote a new one, and handed it to me. "You should probably make an appointment to get established sometime," she said. And walked out.

In the days after the shocks, I slept in fits. I bent over my scorched heart. I stood before the mirror, staring at my flawless skin. There were no marks. If I had been struck by lightning, my chest might have borne the thin branched burns where electricity followed water in the body. But this was an internal strike, a direct hit. No lightning flowers spread like pink trees across my breasts.

Now the anger mounted. My arms were sore from the spasms brought on by electricity, my breasts raw down deep. "It was a misfire," I kept saying aloud, to those who were there that night and those who weren't. But in truth, it was not a misfire; the device had done exactly what it was programmed to do. Even though I had been told by Dr. Oza that I would not be shocked unless my heart rate reached two hundred beats per minute for six beats or more, there had been some other box checked in my software: "if any." *If any* condition for action is met, rather than *if all* conditions are met. In theory, the ICD was advanced enough to know whether my heart's morphology was normal. It shouldn't have been confused by a heart rate pushed high by exercise, a totally normal heartbeat unfolding at 170 beats per minute. But *if any*. My heart rate had stayed above 170 for more than three minutes, the product of a slightly out-of-shape grad student careening around a soccer field in her long underwear and old cleats, and that, apparently, was also a condition specified inside the device's settings. As I watched the guy on the other team who had fallen get up, the battery generated 820 volts of electricity, the capacitor holding it back until it was fully amassed. Then it discharged into the center of my heart.

In the weeks afterward, I stood in coffee shops expecting to be shocked; I rode my bike expecting to be shocked; I warned my first-year writing students of my condition, in case something were to happen at the head of the room. Never mind that the settings had been fixed. I could feel the sensation saved up in my tissues, the burning that would come, the sickening thump, the scream.

Now I understood there existed inside me a machine I could not control, subject to both human and mechanical errors. The part of me that never wanted the device had been reignited and burned steadily. After sepsis I had recognized, finally, that having an ICD implanted did not exempt me from death; after the shocks, I saw for the first time that the ICD could as easily kill me as save me. The promise of being a cyborg was hollow.

I researched how electricity moves through the body: how much it takes to cause permanent cellular damage, how much it takes to kill. I learned that 50 to 60 percent of patients take a shock within the first nine to eleven months of implantation. I learned how lucky I had been: 10 to 20 percent of all internal cardiac defibrillator patients experience what doctors call electrical storms—three or more shocks within a twenty-four-hour period, triggered by the electrical instability of the heart—in their first two years with the device. I learned that in one study, the mean number of shocks in such a "storm" was *seventeen*.

But I also learned that multiple shocks in tight succession nearly always mean malfunction, since one shock should be adequate to disrupt an arrhythmia.

"Multiple shocks [are] the most frightening for patients, causing them to wonder if the device [is] really working or if the ICD [will] even kill them," write Cynthia M. Dougherty and her colleagues in the *Journal of Cardiovascular Nursing*. And, indeed, "any shock increases the chance of cardiac mortality by two-fold....Pathological studies have demonstrated fibrosis and acute cellular injury in the hearts of patients who have had recent shocks." Even single shocks often cause significant psychological aftereffects, including heightened self-monitoring of bodily functions, uncertainty, increased dependence, reactive depression, helplessness, and post-traumatic stress disorder. Dougherty notes that "anxiety scores of those receiving ICD shocks ha[ve] been reported to be similar to those with panic disorder." I would learn, much later, that ICD patients had committed suicide after being shocked.

The medical professionals I'd turned to the morning after had treated my experience as though it were normal, had waved me off as one who carried no wounds. But it struck me that in any other period in history, to take electricity of this kind would mean nothing short of a spiritual transformation; it would signal a sign from the gods. This was lightning from a clear sky. A dark hand reaching down to touch the heart. I couldn't stop thinking about what my insides must look like: the shining twists of burned tissue, thickening, flowers of the body cavity. The way that, when lightning hits ground, sand fuses in long fingers that reach deep into the earth.

I found myself toying with magnets, holding them in the palms of my hands. To place them over the slight rise in my skin would be the easiest way to quiet my cyborg parts, to take back control. But I knew that this was a form of ceding control, too. To allow the arrhythmia—its erratic logic and underlying threat—to inhabit my body unopposed was to lean into death as an inevitable part of the human experience. It was the opposite of my long fight to have the device implanted; it was either spiritually bold or the worst kind of nihilism.

Not long after the shocks, I received the bill for my first device check under my new graduate-student insurance. In Colorado, the device checks had cost $30, the price of a specialist copay. The bill I received in Tucson was for $675. I understood that my new insurance had a fresh deductible, but I understood, too—having worked the back end of a clinic—that this was likely a coding error, a matter of which umbrella the simple ten-minute visit fell under. I called and called. Over the years since I passed out in Jackson, I'd become forceful on these calls, spitting my words, growing loud. I knew that the people on the other end were humans, far removed from the decision makers, but I knew also that they held an inordinate power over my financial life and therefore my body—over the way I stalled or not on necessary health-care visits. "A device interrogation is not a procedure," I shouted at the phone when the billing agent told me how the visit had been coded.

"Jesus himself could not change this coding!" the woman said. Never mind that Jesus himself did not, to my knowledge, ever present Lazarus with an itemized bill.

I wanted it out of me. I dreamed of the magnets as a way of absolving myself of the requirement that I maintain it in any way, of the requirement that I prostrate myself to a system that so clearly did not care for me. I could die anyway. In the end, the bill was resubmitted, and $675 somehow became $275, and I put that $275 on a credit card just before it would have gone to collection, my graduate-school stipend unaccommodating to such sudden bills. The $275 that I paid for the pacer clinic to download a few month's fruitless observations off my ICD could, I calculated, have bought me eighteen appointments at the community acupuncture clinic that had proved essential to restrengthening my parasympathetic nervous system. There, practitioners placed a gentle hand against my wrist to listen to my pulse, asked how I was, and listened carefully. They were people with whom I had built real relationships, reciprocal and empathetic, and who lay soft blankets over my body while I rested. Arguing down the cost of the bill had saved me $400 by one measure, but I could feel inside me the accumulation of these conversations, the quickening escalation, the full-body nausea when the bills arrived in the mail. I was paying in other ways. I knew the precise difference between having insurance and not having insurance, of course, but most of the time that difference was invisible, seemingly meaningless.

One of the central lies of modern health care, I realized then, was that it was doctors and facilities that bestowed good health upon us. That it was my visits and payments, my total compliance, that somehow added up to health.

My life had been saved by IV antibiotics. My treatment plan during sepsis had been built by blood cultures and a battery of high-tech scans. I'd had pictures of my heart taken down my throat, which would have saved my life had the infection moved into my wires. I knew precisely the value of modern medicine. And yet I knew also that you could pump a person full of antibiotics and still lose her. There was some vitality that a body had or didn't have, allowing it to respond to treatments or not—a fire that burned or went out. That vitality did not come from doctors. Perhaps it could, but it was far from reliant on them, and it could certainly be weakened by them. Each time I sustained the injury of being assigned a treatment inappropriate for my stage of life, each time I was treated as irrational or invisible, my opinion irrelevant to my own care—each time I fought about a bill— it adversely affected my well-being.

At the same time, there were things my body knew, essential to health, that were so often overlooked. I thought about the night I'd been sent home from the ER septic, terrified, begging them not to discharge me. And how that night on the soccer field, in the midst of taking two thousand volts to my heart, some critical intelligence had told me, *You can either scream or breathe.* Without it, there would have been a fourth shock, then a fifth, maybe a sixth before the effect of the exercise wore off and my heart tipped below 170 beats per minute. I had more power over my health than I'd ever understood, and what I couldn't control would hardly be helped by my paying hundreds of dollars for visits that told me nothing.

I quietly quit having my device checked.

CAUSA MATERIALIS
CHAPTER 11

Fort Dauphin, Madagascar
2014

I f you trace the island down its eastern seaboard from the port of Toamasina, just before its end you will come across a series of long half-moons of coast framed by peninsulas that jut out like misshapen feet. The town of Taolagnaro—still popularly known by its French colonial name, Fort Dauphin—forms a messy web between two of them, hemmed into a narrow corridor between the ocean and the foothills of the Anosienne, black cliffs velvet with green. The northern moon is Shipwreck Bay; the southern, Libanona Bay.

In the curving belly of Libanona Bay sits the Port d'Ehoala. By the time I arrived in June of 2014, the port had been dredged. A long jetty of white stones broke water for the wharfs. Beside the dock sat a warehouse, a shipping container yard, a raised belt for loading, and orange container cranes with webbed steel sides. The quay was suitable for cruise ships, those big layer cakes of white metal and windows that crossed the Mozambique Channel from Durban.

Oil arrived at the Port d'Ehoala, along with cheap rice, cars, and shipping containers of supplies from international aid groups. What went out was scrap metal, mica, spiky purple lychee, crayfish, vegetable oil, fresh fish, and sisal.

But mostly what went out was the ilmenite and zircon.

Just behind the port, atop a stubby black rise, the land still bore the marks of those who'd lived there: faint trails through the brush, timber cut in wide swaths. But the people were paid in cash to move up the spit, into small blue houses with metal roofs. And the fishermen who spent days casting their nets in Libanona Bay in wooden pirogues were given boats of fiberglass, boats with engines, so they could roam into parts of the ocean that had more fish, though the fishermen would tell me they got far fewer boats from the mining company than they needed, and that many of them joined the strike that blocked the road to the mine.

In any event, the port was appropriately isolated: open for business.

Just inland lay the airport, and south of there, the quarry: another mountain missing its face. What was once mountain became the road, became the thin piles of riprap in Libanona Bay—the two ears that kept sand from slipping away. This was all a World Bank project—the port and the road—in coordination with the Madagascar government and the mine. In town, the muddy back roads were now squared cobblestone, which gleamed in the rain but did not run. A neat asphalt highway ran between the quarry and the port and on through town toward the mine.

If you looked closely at this coast you would see sand swirled dark with what looked like dirt or ash. You'd see it in the places dunes poured out of the grass. You'd see it under your feet as you walked barefoot beside the water. This black wash: this was the metal.

The road to Mandromondromotra was bad.

"Dude," I said as a three-foot-deep red hole passed to our right. My interpreter, Tina, grinned, carefully angling the wheel of the truck, a shiny red Nissan we'd rented from his uncle. A slender man with a round nose and a head of curls, Tina had been so quiet on the day we'd met that I wasn't sure if he liked me. But his English seemed solid; he was the boyfriend of a British NGO employee, and he'd worked with researchers and film crews in this area. Now that we were out of town, he seemed to be lightening up.

"That is a very bad one," he said, smirking.

It was the protest that had snared me, months before, showing up in my searches as I made preparations to visit Ambatovy up north.

147

To study the potential bright side of mining was interesting. But was I really going to go all the way to Madagascar and not travel to the south, where there had been *a protest*? Particularly when the mine in question produced ilmenite, the mineral that becomes titanium?

I had a titanium can at the top of my left breast. I had to visit.

The mineral sands project, QIT Madagascar Minerals—known locally as QMM and owned 80 percent by the Anglo-Australian mining giant Rio Tinto and 20 percent by the government of Madagascar—is a high-quality ilmenite deposit in Fort Dauphin that, if fully exploited, would account for nearly 10 percent of the world market, at seventy million tonnes. Created with an investment of $940 million, QMM had been the first large industrial project of its kind in Madagascar. Construction began in January of 2006. The ilmenite extracted there, I learned upon arrival, would be purified into titanium dioxide concentrate or titaniferous slag, the vast majority of which would become titanium pigment, the high-quality white painted on our walls or dotted on our toothbrushes. The global market chewed through titanium white, while a much smaller percentage of the concentrate went to titanium metal producers for the aerospace industry, artificial hips, and, of course, defibrillator cans.

In reports about the protest, I read that locals carrying spears and slingshots blocked 200 workers, including the chief executive, inside the QMM site, protesting the low prices paid for their land back in 2006. In 2011 a group of around a thousand villagers had filed a class-action lawsuit in UK courts, but the lawsuit was dismissed after the company settled with so many of them that too few litigants remained. On the day of the protest they were also demanding that more locals be hired. In town, I'd heard that although the mine officially hired mostly locals, a certificate of residency was easy to come by; that some of the people supposedly "local" to Anosy—one of Madagascar's twenty-two regions—looked remarkably like the Merina, an ethnic group in the highlands, who traditionally lived around Antananarivo. I'd heard rumors of people paying for access to the rare positions at the mine. How much truth existed in any of these charges was unclear, but the rumors themselves seemed an expression of the ways the mine had disrupted the town. With the opening of QMM, hotels sold out for two years, collapsing the tourism business. The flow of sex workers and mining money into the area spiked sexually transmitted infection rates. And, of course, the cost of living increased.

We'd followed the glossy black asphalt highway through downtown and then out toward the mountains, in the narrow space between the foothills and the sea. It was the best road I'd traveled in Madagascar, until it wasn't. It seemed we had gone off the edge of the world, the red dirt rising and falling in crazy, craterlike ruts. At best we bumped along on washboard. We passed men riding bikes with giant precarious sacks of charcoal strapped behind their seats, thick black sticks poking out the end of the bundles. *There goes the forest,* I couldn't help thinking.

"The mining company only builds the sections that benefit them," Tina said of the road, which at the moment, with my eyeballs rattling in my head, seemed a gross injustice.

Later, I would see photos of the area from above. Along the eastern edge of Route Nationale 12A, to our right, a dark green patch stood out starkly against the light green and red mosaic around it. This, I realized, was the Mandena Conservation Zone, run by the mine. We'd stopped in the village of Nahampoana along the way, and heard how they'd lost access to the forest there; that guards and cameras monitored the area. In the photos, Mandena looked deep and dense, yet so very small beside the rest of the plucked landscape.

On the way to Mandromondromotra, the mountains wore their remaining forest like dark little hats. They bulged with black marbled cliffs. Tina and I rumbled over bridges beside glinting rice paddies. We passed through grassy, sandy open spaces where I could see dark swirls of ilmenite mixed into the white grains; we passed the northern entrance to the mining property, where the road got good again.

In the center of Mandromondromotra, men and women sat outside a small wooden shop. One side of the shop displayed full shelves of Three Horses and Castel beer; on the other, a woman cooked over a charcoal fire. A man leaned into the kitchen to light his cigarette from the coals.

"In vaovao?" Tina asked, meaning: What's the news? He reached

forward to shake the hands of the men, explaining who we were, asking to talk with them about their experiences since the mine went in.

Oil was in the rice field, they said. Part of the field would not grow. When the wind blew from the mine, they felt ill. They got fevers, headaches. Banana trees that used to give fruit now produced just a few. Though they looked ripe, they were not.

The national government got the money, they said. They didn't know what the local government had done with its share.

A man in a blue windbreaker leaned forward, peeling small oranges, dropping the peels into a plastic bag at his feet. The peels were pale, almost yellow, green in places. *Does the wind have a different smell from normal? Did the water look normal where the rice did not grow? Can I see?* Either Tina did not understand my questions, or no one understood him.

When Tina said, "People are giving birth to things which are not babies," I assumed there was a translation problem.

The woman who said it was squatting, dressed in a faded navy-blue quilted jacket, her hair in buns. She rocked back and forth as she spoke.

"When a girl has a baby," Tina said. "It is not complete." The feet were warped or missing, he said. There were no ears. There were missing fingers or toes. "It looks like the inside of an egg. If a baby, the head is really big. Or they don't have a part of body." The woman jabbed her finger into the air.

"Tina, are we talking about miscarriage here?" He looked at me blankly. "You know, when a pregnancy fails? The baby dies inside the woman or the woman gives birth too early?"

He shrugged. "She does say the woman gives birth at six months sometimes."

I nodded, unsettled. "Did this happen before the mine went in?"

Tina conferred with the woman, who grabbed one of the oranges and peeled it in a single movement. "When QMM start the mining, they have that problem," he said.

She was trying to say something about babies needing sun, but Tina's translations fell apart: "Baby need sun. Baby doesn't have enough sun, doctor says this. One hour. When they're sleeping. It's not enough time to sleep," he said, and my head spun; was it Tina or the stories being told that didn't make sense? I tried to parse what they meant, what questions to ask to make the situation clear.

But he went on, for the crowd was growing, and with it the tension of many people wanting to speak. "They don't have papers for their land. But the land is grandpa and grand and grand. This is one hundred, two hundred years ago. They say, there is a 2005 law. If you have land you have to be working on the land. But we sometimes leave fallow," said Tina. "And the government gives a lawyer to take land by force."

"They need a solution because they feel hurt by the mine," Tina said.

"Are you surprised by what we heard?" I asked Tina later, down the rutted road, headed for a fishing village. I could feel my heart in my throat.

He paused. "Not much," he said.

"I am," I told him. The horror of what we had been told lodged in my belly. *People are giving birth to things which are not babies.*

But what did it *mean*? What was causing it? Ilmenite extraction, as far as I knew, was a process without chemicals; the company separated sands using magnets and gravity. In some of the other villages, and in the market, people had talked about an increase in malaria, about dizziness and fevers and itching, people falling down and dying, and yet this didn't match the process I'd read about. "Some of those descriptions were a little hard to swallow," I said to Tina, and even I could hear my voice grow tinny. Things happened for *reasons*, I told him. Of course I wanted to believe the villagers, but I needed more information; I wasn't an epidemiologist.

Tina drove without expression, without response.

In the United States, I told him archly, we were very scientific. Just because we suspected something was true did not mean it was. "Their pain is real," I said. But what actually caused it? Had the rates of fevers and miscarriages and malaria actually risen? Or were they just on high alert for the potential damages of a project that broke their hearts? And if the rates *had* risen, what drove the increase? Was it something like immune suppression, from the despair of losing their forests? Did dust play a role? Were there more standing pools of water for mosquito breeding? What, of these, could cause such deformations?

The whole drive back I twitched with urgency: I needed to find someone whose job it was to quantify this, to talk through it, to point me toward the research that would tell me if this was real.

The babies were born like the insides of an egg.

The babies were born missing their limbs.

We absolutely did not know, I told Tina, that the cause of any of this was Rio Tinto.

From the entrance of the hotel, the infinity pool lay a short walk down steep wooden steps. The pool was a long white rectangle with a shallow section at its end jutting off like a *p,* the water the most absolute blue I'd ever seen. At the bungalow bar, tables waited in the shade, the liquor shelf stocked full. A thick green cushion the size of a full mattress sat next to the deep end of the pool on a raised wood frame, looking out over the ocean. Presumably this was for lovers, honeymooners pulling themselves from the water and collapsing together in the sun.

Each day I traveled into places where people did not have enough to eat, then returned here. Again I'd booked a hotel I knew would have decent Wi-Fi and an English-speaking concierge; these were the basics that made my work possible, with my limited experience and only five and a half weeks on the island. This hotel, on the sunset side of the peninsula, cost $50 a night, a fortune for Madagascar but absurdly cheap considering my balcony, which dangled out over a steep hillside, shielded by mango and eucalyptus trees, curving tastefully away from the other rooms. From there I could see the sea foam violently over the reef in Libanona Bay, and the misted-over face of Pic St. Louis rising sharply 1,735 feet above the ocean.

In the mornings I crouched with my notebook on my knee in a fishing village beside the hanging carcasses of zebu, or I ducked into a corner store to talk to a small business owner as she scooped flour into to-go sacks for customers. I tried to hold my eye contact steady as I wrote, as I quietly asked Tina to have them elaborate, trying to make each person feel seen. Yet in late afternoon, as I slipped into the infinity pool to swim laps, the sense I'd had all trip that we existed in different worlds became suffocating. Although I had come here to see the mark of metal, in many ways I had more in common with the mining companies than the people who bore the brunt. I had been raised inside their capitalist logic, in the world of efficiency, assessments, contracts, and white papers. I was the literal daughter of corporate America. Here I was, qualifying my statements, seeking an expert to validate what I'd been told. The mine's social responsibility employees, drinking Three Horses beer on the hotel porch with the rest of the expats, could have been my friends at home, returned from the Peace Corps, graduates of top master's programs in international development. And if I went into cardiac arrest on that porch, I knew that the beer drinkers would help whisk me to better medical care than any of the villagers I'd spoken to could access. I had arrived on the island with some hope that my voice could amplify the experience of these communities. Yet for all the repetition of their losses, I didn't know what their connection to the land actually felt like, what health meant in their lives. And in all likelihood, the people I interviewed had no frame of reference for what a defibrillator is; I didn't tell them what had brought me.

In 2019, I would read that a full five countries in Africa have no cardiologist at all and that half the countries on the continent lack a single cardiac catheterization lab. (The study did not include Madagascar, which means either there are no cardiologists in the country, the Pan-African Society of Cardiology isn't yet connected with them, or that practitioners didn't answer the survey.) In high-income areas such as the United States, Canada, and western Europe, pacemakers are implanted at a rate of between 300 and 1,200 per million people, according to a 2018 *Heart Rhythm Journal* article, while in sub-Saharan Africa the rate falls between one and seven per million, despite higher rates of heart disease because of parasite-related arrhythmias and scarring from early-life rheumatic fevers. These are pacemaker and not ICD rates, because pacemakers are viewed as life-sustaining—whereas ICDs for most people, including me, are considered prophylactic. ICDs are rare on the continent outside of a few major surgery centers, clustered mostly in northern African nations and in South Africa. In many villages, I'd read, cardiac events were likely to be considered spiritual events—caused by witchcraft—rather than medical ones. Autopsies were rarely performed; an arrhythmia as technical as long QT would likely never be diagnosed, considering the technologies required for a workup. Far more than cardiac care, the people I interviewed needed access to birth control, antimalarials, and burn care for children who fell in the cooking fires; they lived with tuberculosis, maternal mortality, and worms.

I hadn't come to Madagascar to document health inequity, but it was impossible not to think about, given what *had* brought me. But perhaps most maddening of all was that the majority of titaniferous slag wasn't headed for defibrillator cans and artificial hips; it was headed onto our *toothbrushes* in a little blob. If people were giving birth to things that were not babies, and if the reason was an ilmenite mine, the question was not whether I should get another defibrillator. The question was whether we should still find it appropriate to paint our walls titanium white.

I didn't expect the mine to be beautiful. On the drive from QMM's downtown interpretive center to the plant, low swoops of dunes unfolded around us, patches of white sand glowing in the golden afternoon light. Here and there dry grasses held the hillsides. Some of the road cuts were a searing white, shaped by wind, as though we'd wandered into an avalanche zone in the dead of winter. In others, the topsoil had mixed with the sand when they took out the trees, and now in the smooth, shaved landscape, dark swirls made it look as though we were driving through a giant bowl of cookies-and-cream ice cream.

In places the sand was cluttered by dense little stands of banana, coconut, and eucalyptus, with steep little ravines eroded between them, the forest floor rowdy with green shoots. Aimé—my tour guide, a tall man in a smart gray button-down, fashionable glasses, and a pair of hiking boots—told me that the presence of these species was a sign that this was actually secondary forest. The rare littoral forest people spoke so much about—a specialized humid forest adapted to sand, rich with endemic species, and believed to have stretched more than 1,600 kilometers down Madagascar's eastern coast—had been harvested long ago, he said, with the locals planting high densities of these crop trees in their place. Even the conservation area, he said, was technically secondary forest.

"When people say there is a forest that will be destroyed, this is it," Aimé said. But my chest still clenched when I saw the little clumps of roots from the disappeared overburden left behind in the sand. As of 2006, when the mine construction began, the Missouri Botanical Garden—a nonprofit organization particularly active in documenting Madagascar's endemic species—noted that just 10.3 percent of Madagascar's original littoral forest still existed, in isolated chunks, and that 535 hectares of it was located at Mandena. Another 835 hectares remained at Petriky, to the south of Libanona Bay, and yet another 1,580 hectares at Sainte Luce, to the north of Shipwreck Bay. Both sites were slated for exploitation by QMM in the future.

At the Fasimainty Centre in town, Aimé told me that this mine was not really "the mining mold." "We're not digging," he said. "We're just taking sand." He cupped his hand and made a scraping motion. "Like with cake you just take the cream."

He was right: this was not a yawning pit but a man-made lake, repeatedly filled in and moved. After it removed the overburden, QMM would identify a dense deposit, create a hole, and insert its "wet plant": a dredge and high-pressure hose connected to an initial processing plant that sat in the water. The hose would shoot water at the banks of the pit at high pressure, crumbling the sand into the water. The dredge then sucked this sand-water combination up and into the wet plant, where the slurry ran through a series of spirals that separated the ilmenite from the rest of the sand by gravity. The rejected sand shot out the back of the wet plant, while the ilmenite moved through another pipe to a waiting area away from the man-made lake, outside the main suppression plant, where—after four to five days of drying—a bulldozer pushed heaps of the black mineral up a conveyor belt. Inside the main suppression plant, the zircon and titanium were separated by magnets.

"No chemicals, just physics," Aimé said.

"Really? No chemicals?"

"The engineer is useful sometimes," he said, smiling.

The sun dipped low. The smoke from *tavy* and charcoal production was settling, becoming long blue feathers at the base of the mountain. Aimé had the driver take a left toward the treed section he'd pointed out on our way in, the portion of its lease QMM didn't cut: the Mandena Conservation Zone. We passed the curve of a reclamation zone, where the sand had been reheaped and planted with saplings, their skinny bodies sticking out of white plastic covering.

We passed an employee soccer field. Then a wetland. The forest thickened.

Then all at once it opened back up, and we were inside an enormous nursery. On both sides of the road sat long rows of raised tables, covered in seedlings in small plastic bags. Above them, irrigation tubing dripped, strapped to a grid of long wooden poles. Everything smelled like water.

One side, Aimé showed me, was all endemic species—the ones inventoried by the mine before Mandena was stripped, which they would use in reclamation. On the other side of the road grew nonnative species, mostly fast-growing trees like eucalyptus, which would help meet the villagers' needs for wood sooner.

"We're still finding new species," Aimé said. "We have sixty-five endemic species here." He added, "This area, not in Madagascar— this area." He smiled. "Just last month we found a new one and gave it the CEO's name."

"We can walk for a moment?" Aimé said. "Just a short way." I nodded.

The road past the nursery was sand and dirt, and the trees pushed in against it, their foliage hanging over the path. When we'd lost sight of the car, Aimé stopped me. "Listen," he said, and at first I thought something was wrong. Then he smiled. "Can you hear the silence?"

I heard crickets, the sound of shifting birds, the rasp of leaves brushing leaves. Beneath it, yes, silence. A yawn of quiet. Something deep in me relaxed.

Aimé told me he came camping here when he was stressed. I thought for a moment that I would like that, before the faces of the villagers in Nahampoana flickered across my mind. Kept out by guards and cameras. As the forest darkened, we began walking again. The place seemed impossibly dense. "So this has not been inhabited in a while," I said, and even as I said it I was thinking of my home country. How the places I camped—the "untouched" forests I adored, the public land protected from mining—had also been taken from indigenous people.

"Yes," he said. "Not since"—he looked up—"2002."

"Wow. So it has been regrowing for a decade."

"Yes."

"Would it look like this? If people had been allowed in?"

Aimé looked at me squarely. "No." We walked in silence for a minute. "Here," he said finally, "all the stress fall down."

He told me people used to look at the mountains and see trees. "Now we can see stone on the mountain." He told me he knew tourists found the dramatic view appealing—and I laughed because it was true, I loved the long gray cliffs—but their visibility was a product of deforestation. Ten years ago, he said, there was a meter of soil covering that mountain. Now it was gone, along with the trees. What remained was this scrap—an area, I read later, smaller than Brooklyn's Prospect Park.

From space astronauts have said it looks like the island is bleeding to death—her red soils pouring into the ocean. The result of *tavy*, of logging for charcoal and the illegal rosewood trade, of desertification and erosion.

When I'd flown over, it looked like someone had peeled back the scalp of the land.

We passed a browned trunk on the side of the trail—shoulder-high, a husk of a plant—and Aimé went to it. He sighed. Sometimes they tried to replant the trees they removed from the mine site, establishing them here in Mandena, and this plant was one of those. He shrugged as if to say, Clearly it doesn't always work. This one, he told me, was a cousin of the banana, a plant that made bright rubbery fruit sometimes used in villages to feed pigs.

We stopped at the bridge, leaning our elbows onto its wooden railing. Eucalypti near the water shed their skin in soft spirals. The river poured over smooth stones, eating at a couple of old logs that had landed in the flow. Bats ducked over us. Aimé told me the conservation area got three thousand visitors annually, that if I were in town longer I could take a canoe down this river—a sultry journey through the heart of Mandena.

"We could walk and walk and walk!" Aimé said, throwing his arms into the air. "But it will be night." He nodded at me to follow him back.

"So in forty years," I said slowly, "the mine site will look like this?"

"That's the idea," he said.

And with a shock I realized I believed him.

As we approached the truck, he thanked me. "This was good even for me," he said.

On the drive back to town, Aimé talked.

"It is very hard," he said. "Normally, without the mine, there would be no forest here. The forest are savings for the people. Each time they have a difficulty, they take trees to get money. They will say, since the time of my grandfathers there has always been forest. How are you to say it will disappear?" He shook his head. "They always use natural resources as their primary resource.

"The forests are in danger here. Not from the mine but from the people." The mining zone, he said, destroyed six thousand hectares for fifty years, but it would rehabilitate these lands after. He asked me to compare this to the community, which destroyed five thousand hectares per year, indefinitely, without rehabilitating it. "The problem in Madagascar is not really the people. It is the poverty. If the government can tackle poverty, they could think about conserving the forest. With more education they can know it is important to conserve for their grandson.

"We have many resources. The problem is management. We could have ten Rio Tintos, but if there's no accountability, we will remain poor. There are fifty thousand people here. Maybe two thousand working for the mine in some way. The benefit will not come from the employment. It will come from the royalties. If the government doesn't play its role, it will not be efficient. We need many parties to make it work. To make the magic happen. But I do believe it's feasible."

Then, as the driver turned onto a dirt road, Aimé pointed out across Shipwreck Bay. "Look!" he said. Just inland from the shore lay a small line of lights. "That's where we just were. That's the dredge."

As we began to rise up the peninsula toward my hotel, I kept craning my head back, to see those lights like beacons. To see where sand turned to metal.

Less than two years later, Rio Tinto, which owned 80 percent of QMM—with its bottom line suffering after a bad investment in Mozambique—would dissolve its corporate environmental mandate for a "Net Positive Impact," which required that its ecosystem improvements outpace biodiversity losses. By the time the mandate lifted, Rio Tinto had fallen behind in its restoration activities in southeastern Madagascar, not increasing forest cover enough to offset damage from its mining operations. The pressure from loggers and charcoal producers had grown, with forest loss spiking in the two sites they'd intended to treat like Mandena, preserving the most intact forest fragments and mining the rest—Sainte Luce and Petriky. Rio Tinto's official new environmental policy focused on "minimizing residual impact"—a vague and toothless standard that led to the resignation of all but one of the researchers serving on QMM's biodiversity committee.

Less than five years later, a UK-based NGO called the Andrew Lees Trust released two independent studies showing that mining activity on the Mandena concession had trespassed into a lake that should have been legally protected by an eighty-meter buffer. While a background level of radioactivity was always present in the sands of this area, industrial processes like removing ilmenite can disrupt their secular equilibrium, increasing the concentration of radioactive elements. It's believed that tailings from Mandena were used to build the berm separating the mining processes from the lake— waste sand containing uranium-238, thorium-232, and their decay products (including other radionuclides such as radium-226). Although the researchers did not believe radioactive tailings had yet entered local drinking-water sources, the scientists who completed the study worried about one of the region's frequent cyclones causing overflow into the lake or raising the water table enough for seepage to occur. After more than two years of claiming they'd complied with all legally mandated buffers, in March of 2019 Rio Tinto finally released a memo admitting to the breach, which they called "unintended." While the company suggests the breach occurred in 2014–2015, a study commissioned by Rio Tinto itself in 2018 from the Australian consultancy Ozius Spatial suggests that by early 2014—before my arrival—the company had already encroached onto the lake bed.

Perhaps I believed Aimé that day because he lived in my world: the one in which we drank cocktails on the porch of nice hotels, attended university, and relocated for jobs. The one in which we benefited from metal. Perhaps I believed him because he was speaking my language. Perhaps I believed him because I wanted to—because the only thing making mining on this island palatable was a belief that the involvement of multinational corporations would provide the necessary—and otherwise unavailable—resources to restore habitat in such a rare and powerful place. Perhaps I believed him because I'd conveniently forgotten that the forest at Mandena had not only been allowed to grow for ten years while protected from use, it had also never suffered the violence of first being stripped of its overburden and mined. I had forgotten the sad transplanted tree whose roots didn't take. The saplings QMM would place in those smooth sandy bowls of ice cream—in the barren open—would have to muster a resilience no older forest like the Mandena Conservation Zone ever needed.

Perhaps I believed Aimé because it had become painfully clear that, no matter how many years of life I gained from an implanted cardiac defibrillator—if any at all, given the sepsis and the shocks and whatever else came next—there was not a thing I could do with myself, not even over the course of a lifetime, that would be worth what it had cost.

And perhaps because—even if I went without a defibrillator for the rest of my life—I wouldn't want my sister told no.

PART II
THE DISMANTLING

CHAPTER 12

Tucson, Arizona
2016

At first I thought there was something wrong with the plane. The humming was subtle and steady, there in the air above Lake Erie, with a few skinny islands slipping into the fog beneath us. My friend Melisa and I were en route to Bogotá, Colombia, for a week of mountain biking, hiking, and wine sipping in broad cobblestone plazas. Melisa, a middle school teacher, was on spring break, the flights were cheap, and the dollar was strong against the peso.

Is it the engine? I thought, looking around.

Then I put a hand to my chest.

The life of a cyborg unfolds like this, with strange mechanical things happening to my body, and me always a step behind. Then I understood: *low battery.* I grabbed Melisa's hand, pressed it to the rise on my chest. "Feel this," I said, and her eyes widened. I would have three months.

By then it had been six and a half years since implantation, four since the ICD accidentally shocked me on that soccer field, and nearly two since I'd come home from Madagascar. However the quest to determine whether I would get another device had shaped my life, I understood what I had been gifted in that respite of years. On a daily level, I had forgotten the ICD's existence. It had settled into my body. I ran eight-mile trail races. I slept on my belly. While I could theoretically go into cardiac arrest, I traveled believing I wouldn't. I had hiked the long muddy road to Maroseranana despite its complete lack of cell service, clinics, or CPR-certified strangers.

Every ICD is programmed to vibrate when it crosses below a certain battery threshold. I had, in theory, known this was coming. At the start of the year, I had pored over my insurance options, running the calculations. If the surgery to replace the device arrived this year and I met my deductible and coinsurance, how much would it cost me on this plan? On that plan? Should I opt for the low premium and low specialist copays but the high deductible, assuming this wouldn't be the year?

But even though I ran the calculations, I thought I would have longer. They'd told me the battery could last eight years at implantation. I'd only ever been shocked that one night. In November, my parents had flown out to Colorado to be with Christine for her replacement procedure on the Wednesday before Thanksgiving. In my mind, she should have been a full year ahead of me. As it was, her techs helped her run down her battery through extra pacing so she could ensure her replacement procedure fell just before the end of 2015 and not after; she had funds in a health savings account that wouldn't roll over at the new year.

"Disease interrupts a life," writes the socionarratologist Arthur Frank, "and illness then means living with perpetual interruption."

I had forgotten that my experience would cross again into unknown territory, that the story I told as finished would be reopened. That there would be hospitals. That there would be new room for things to go very wrong.

Now, with the machine's second buzz, a cold fear swept into my body. I knew what my life was about to become.

It was March 12, 2016. I had three months of battery life. But at the beginning of June, I would head to Tanzania to begin a summer job working with teens in a global leadership program, and I knew better than to take any open incisions with me to the African continent. I'd need to leave a buffer period in case anything went wrong; I'd need to undergo the procedure in April, in a little over a month.

What lay before me was complicated mostly because I'd just switched insurance providers and didn't yet have an electrophysiologist. My first year out of graduate school, I'd qualified for Medicaid, benefiting from the Affordable Care Act's expansion of the program to adults with incomes under 133 percent of the federal poverty line. In my second year out, I was earning enough to bump up a level, qualifying for a federally subsidized plan. While it still seemed like a miracle to be able to buy insurance on the Affordable Care Act's marketplace at all, I hadn't realized how limited my options would be. Only one insurer participated in Pima County's exchange, and the electrophysiologist I'd seen in graduate school at University Medical Center would no longer be in network. I'd have to establish with a new primary-care physician first—I was waiting for an appointment, since she was so booked up with new Obamacare clients—then get referred to a new EP, at a different hospital.

What never rose up in me, I noticed right away, was resistance. As I called my new primary-care doctor from Colombia to set up the referral. As I returned to town and met my new cardiologist as soon as I could. As I put a surgery date on the calendar and rescheduled classes that fell too close. Never did I find myself standing in a room, holding the phone, wondering what I was doing. Feeling like I should stop.

Two years earlier, on the way home from Madagascar, I'd spent most of an afternoon on a Ferris wheel overlooking Johannesburg, staring at the tailing piles that dotted the city. It was a quick layover I'd taken knowing the city was considered the mining capital of South Africa and that it headquartered some of the world's largest mining companies. Jo'burg was established in 1886 after prospectors struck gold; when that gold reef was revealed to be the largest in the world, town boomed. By the 1890s, Johannesburg was the most populous city in Africa, with tens of thousands of residents. Thirty-five percent of all gold ever mined came from that area, and the ground was rich in diamonds and platinum, too.

The Ferris wheel sat atop a gold mine that had closed in 1971, part of a theme park called Gold Reef City that I'd found hilarious in concept. Never before had I been able to ride the flying swings, eat an ice cream cone, and hop into a 250-foot mining shaft with helmet and headlamp, all in succession. But it was late June, winter on the Highveld, with the warmth of the sun dimmed by brown haze. After the rainy forests and quiet villages of Madagascar, Jo'burg felt harsh to me. The theme-park screams of people on the Runaway Train seemed hollow. All around me was metal, or money made from metal. Somewhere in the city, platinum miners were engaged in the longest strike in Jo'burg history over their low wages, despite record profits in the industry. Six-lane freeways curved flawlessly around the city. The grocery stores nearest my host's apartment were located deep in gleaming silver shopping malls with five-star hotels and paid underground parking. In South Africa, as elsewhere on the continent, colonial rulers had once used taxes to force rural men out of sub-sistence activities and into the economy. Thousands of men left their families to work in the mines near Jo'burg in order to pay what they "owed," living in single-sex compounds with concrete bunk beds and bare walls, signing contracts that, if broken, left them with a criminal record. The conditions were rough and the hours long, and plenty of men never returned home—dying instead of tuberculosis, silicosis, malnutrition, or from accidents.

The city was made of their accumulated labor, I understood, yet the descendants of these black workers from the "reserves" were likely not the people living in the leafy, walled estates of wealthy Jo'burg suburbs like Houghton. Even now, nearly thirty years after the close of apartheid, black South Africans largely live in a different country from their white counterparts because of the deep accumu-lated wealth gap. In 2014, when I visited, nearly a quarter of the city was unemployed. Thousands of residents still lived in shantytowns. Jo'burg was a city of walls, guards in navy-blue uniforms, barbed wire. The skyscrapers, I thought, might as well be gravestones.

Beneath the Ferris wheel, in the quiet shafts that sunk toward the center of the earth, acid mine water had slowly begun rising, with the possibility of flooding the park if the situation were left unattended. The year before my visit, the park suspended mine tours and moved the museum above ground (although the situation seemed to have improved since then). From the Ferris wheel, I could see a tailing pile tall as a bluff, with a few trees growing out its top. The erosion furrows at the pile's edge—as at the uranium pit I'd discovered in the center of Wyoming—were deep and devoid of life. Another tailing pile formed a butte above a neighborhood. I knew there were residences built on tailings, that the piles blew arsenic and lead and uranium across the city, and that only well-off neighborhoods had the natural windbreaks of vegetation to cut the toxic dust. Even in a place known for its mining wealth, the mess lay before us, without political will or agreement around how to fix it, and with the burden resting, as always, along fault lines of inequality. In the years to come, some of the tailings would disappear not because of public health concerns, but because the small amount of gold they contained was now, through modern methods, economically recoverable.

The flying swings had given me palpitations, making me physically aware of my heart for the first time in a long time. Now I rode the steady tubs of the Ferris wheel into the sky over and over as a comfort—no deep breathing required—but also because I couldn't stop looking at the city beneath me, wondering what the communities I'd visited in Madagascar would look like in a hundred years. I had expected to land on the island and steadily accrue answers. I had hoped to feel delighted by the way all those activists and researchers over the years had infiltrated corporate policy, shifting the ethics of mining. Instead, as I looked out over a mining town heavy with 120 years of legacy, I felt a sort of despair press down over me.

It was so hard to control the impacts of mining.

The processes of extraction and refining are inherently toxic. They just are. They take apart the land. They break open rock that is only chemically stable while intact, or they distill a mineral for market through wildly noxious processes. And there doesn't seem to be a way to spare people the change that comes barreling into their communities. Maybe protecting people from change isn't a realistic goal— change being, as it is, an inevitable condition of being alive, and one that accompanies the best parts of our lives, too. Even a mountain is born of violence. A mountain is the colonizer of open space. But if change is inevitable, heartbreak without comfort is not. Could we limit projects to those that were truly consensual, approved not only by central governments who stood to benefit but also by the individual communities about to absorb losses? Were tragedy and grief the inevitable bedfellows of industrial projects, or was there a way even beyond all those standards to respect and cushion the communities that took the hit for all of us who benefited?

No matter how many hours I spent trying to wrap my head around the chain of impacts, always there was some other factor, some unintended consequence to attend to, even the most well-intentioned projects spinning them off, and it was hard to picture a corporation—having pledged allegiance to the profit mandate—remaining dynamic enough to stay in step with a community in the long aftermath. In this way, I felt an enormous compassion for some of the bright-eyed employees I'd met, at the hotel bar or in off-the-record meetings. It was easy to look at initiatives and declare what wasn't working; it was so much harder to fix them.

And yet extraction is the fundamental human activity. This much I had learned in Madagascar. Even the villagers, victims of industry, panned the streams for gold and cut trees when they needed them. Resources were constantly being harvested on my behalf, too, only because I sat at the end of a long supply chain, I wasn't so acutely aware of them: every square of toilet paper, every cubic foot of natural gas, every carrot and cow.

For so long, I had assumed I would not get another ICD. It was not lost on me that the answer had come so swiftly, without question. Perhaps it was because between the shocks in 2012 and the low-battery buzz in 2016 the ICD had been so quiet, so benign inside me. It had not added to the calculus against it. Or perhaps the decision came easily because my knowledge of the supply chain had, in some way, schooled me out of the belief that saying no would make any kind of difference. By then I carried a smartphone. My toothpaste still contained titanium white.

I acted out of a kind of numbness, then. To live in an industrial society carries costs. It came down to this: in the face of the forces that made metal, I felt so small. And I wanted to live.

By having the surgery, I understood, I was playing a hand of cards.

I was saying yes to several weeks of restricted mobility as the incision healed and the scar tissue rebuilt. I was saying yes to pain; to the risk of infection; to missed work; to paying around $6,700 between the deductible and coinsurance. To the gamble that something else could go wrong. I was saying yes to resources harvested on my behalf.

All this, in exchange for a titanium insurance plan inside my body. As I marched off to boost my immunizations for my summer job in Tanzania, I could feel more than ever the permission slip the ICD offered me—to run alone, to travel alone, to visit countries that otherwise lacked the medical technology to resuscitate me. I exchanged one risk for another. I exchanged one cost for another.

The previous March, I'd driven nearly nine hundred miles east out of Tucson, across the scrappy beige bottom of New Mexico, through the methane-flaring gas fields of West Texas, to the town of Hamilton in the East Texas hill country. This was the town my family helped "found" in the mid-1800s, one of my male ancestors doing a tour in Stephen Austin's Texas Rangers as they drove Comanche out of the region. I'd come to visit the grave of Lena Proctor Standefer, my great-great-grandmother—the woman we saw as our most probable genetic link, the last known stop in a line of ancestors who'd passed down the mutation. No matter how long I'd considered living without an ICD, I always carried Lena's story with me, the counterweight, the cautionary tale, the pretechnology version of my sister and me. In 1879, Lena was born into a world in which doctors were just beginning to learn that electricity drove the pumping of the heart. The EKG would be invented a few years after her death. If she had ever passed out before the day of her death, in March of 1899—if she'd had warning faints, woken up bleary and paralyzed as I did, suffered strange falls from her bed like Christine—we would never know. There was no emergency number to call, no ambulance to send, no automatic external defibrillator hanging on a nearby wall (as is now standard in airports and schools). Her family members would not have known CPR, and the hospital in town, had she made it there, could not have produced paddles to wake her from cardiac arrest.

In the only pictures we have of her, Lena looks like a child, her face porcelain and round, her hair rolled tightly against the top of her head, ringlets spread down her chest. She had a straight mouth and light eyes, like my father. She'd married at nineteen. She was dead by twenty.

The weather was horrible during Lena's last winter, 1898–1899—the worst on record, a volunteer from the Hamilton County Historical Museum told me. Winter tornadoes touched down near Pottsville. Lena—postpartum, and therefore at high risk for long QT–caused torsades de pointes episodes—would have rocked her baby son, Cecil, by gas lamp, listening to the wind tear at the trees.

Tobacco had failed the first settlers, and so in Hamilton the fields went thigh high with cotton bolls, summers full of the humming of gins down on Pecan Creek. Town turned black with the smoke of the burr furnace, where they burned what was caught in the cotton that was not cotton. There were cottonseed presses to harvest lamplight and rattling grain mills. In the summer, everything was heat, a dripping windless humidity broken by occasional darkening storms. Pecans, blackened with mold, split beneath the boot.

In the center of town square sat the majestic Hamilton County Courthouse, three stories of white limestone brick, narrow arched windows, a set of columns pointed east. All around the courthouse, commerce unfolded. Livestock auctions. A bandstand on the south side that murmured and tossed with music. Farmers met in the dirt of the square to load baled cotton and wagons of hay, most headed twenty miles north to Hico, where there was a railroad stop.

I wanted to be able to picture Lena's life—what it was, exactly, that had been cut short. But despite the best efforts of Kay Overton—a cheerful white-haired volunteer from the museum, who wore a jaunty gray-striped cap—I couldn't locate where Lena and her husband, Henry, lived at the time of her death, in 1899. "The Standefers lived quiet lives," Kay said, shaking her head, flipping through archived newspapers and church bulletins at the museum. "They weren't active in church. They weren't visible in the community." In his obituary, Henry was described as "a quiet, likeable man...who meddled with no one's affairs and demanded the same consideration from other people." In the black-and-white picture of him taken around the time of their wedding, Henry is strikingly handsome, clean-shaven, with a strong jawline, thick neck, and eyes that seem to sparkle despite his straight face.

In the unheated voluminous old warehouse that holds the town's genealogy archives, Kay and I flipped through binders of cemetery records. We found only what we already knew: a listing in the Independent Order of Odd Fellows cemetery a few blocks away for Henry and his second wife, Bertha, with no mention of Lena. Within the hour I stood on the spring earth before Henry's grave. Beside the gray double headstone that bore Henry and Bertha's names lay a white marble slab commemorating their son David—my father's great-half-uncle—who'd died a prisoner of war in Manchuria at the Mukden camp during World War II.

It was David's grave that brought me to my knees—the circumstances of his death, his young age of twenty-three—and only then did I notice that his gravestone was askew, that it had moved and would move. Beneath the white slab of marble sat another stone.

"Sorry, bud," I whispered to David, lifting his gravestone off.

With my hand I cleared mud from the weathered stone beneath, pushing my finger into the grooves flush with cool, wet dirt, carving out what was there. My heart racing. I could feel, then, how acutely I desired not only to know what Lena's life had been like but also her death. I wanted to know the specifics of how she had gone down, whether she was startled by a crash of thunder or the screams of her own infant in the middle of the night, how she fit into our lineage. To know her in some way—to find where her body had been placed into the ground—felt like it had something to tell me, about whether or not I was obligated to like and use this technology, whether my complaints were just those of the privileged.

I sat back on my heels on the lawn.

"Unlike in my dreams, this doesn't say Lena Proctor Standefer," I told Kay, and she laughed. The grooves in the stone were just places it had been worn away by weather. Still, the bottom stone seemed out of place, for as we walked the rows of headstones, plenty of graves from the 1940s resembled David's—the white marble, the same font—yet none of them sat atop another stone. And that worn, mossy, green-black stone resembled the graves of those marked dead between 1890 and 1900.

"Maybe they buried David right on top of her," Kay said. At the time of David's death, Bertha's husband would have been dead four years; maybe she wanted her son right there beside her. Maybe there was no need to keep a grave, forty-four years later, for the first wife, a woman no one mourned anymore.

So it was possible that the body of Lena had been right there. But in that era before embalming, Kay told me, it was equally likely she simply hadn't died in town. If a woman like Lena met her death out on the homestead, visiting her parents-in-law—perhaps staying with them after the birth of the baby—they wouldn't have hauled her back to town decomposing. She would have been laid to rest right there.

Which meant her body might be on old Standefer land.

The fence was an easy one—a white steel-tube stock gate, fastened with a snap chain. I climbed the metal bars, set my foot squarely on the chain loop, and propelled myself over, quickly crossing the two-track to duck into the cedars along the property line. My heart yammered. Beta-blockers excepted, I've never been good at breaking the rules.

All around me, the hills of central Texas tilted down toward the Leon River, their tops brown with early spring. All of the farms were fallow. A week ago, there'd been snow. Now the sun shone through a gauzy layer of clouds, tall grass concealing bunched prickly pear.

What I was looking for could be anywhere: one of those old corners with slumping outbuildings, rusted parts, some grown-over family cemetery with humble marker stones. The evidence of lives lived on this land. Neither the original Standefer deed Kay and I retrieved from the county clerk's office nor the GIS map the appraiser's office printed off showed where the houses had been then.

An eight-foot-tall welded-wire deer fence kept me from hiking into the northeastern flank of old Standefer land. It looked climbable, but I worried over a twisted ankle, over heavily armed Texans. I walked beside the fence, on the kind of dull trail formed by cattle or white-tail, staring off through the wire boxes to see what I could of the rest of the land: just a dirt road and more scrubland.

I followed the slope of the land toward the river. In dry washes I found exposed flanks of limestone. I found tangles of skinny trees, bright patches of green where water recently ran.

Henry left the baby somewhere on this land with his parents. He went off somewhere we don't know. Henry wouldn't marry again for fifteen years. However invisible this woman seemed now, she left her marks on a man.

Down at the Leon River I stepped onto the strung and exposed roots of a tree, descending them like a rope ladder onto the steep muddy banks. Then I took off my shoes and waded in.

The place was silent but for the creak of the trees and the sweet pulse of water, occasional insects. I could imagine what it would have been like for Lena in the final summer of her life, pregnant, how this forest had thickened, how the mosquitoes clustered densely along the river. I imagined what a relief this stretch of land at her in-laws' would have been after the noise of town, with its buzzing cotton gins and reams of thick black smoke running out of the burr furnace.

I understood then that there would be no grave. What I wanted of Lena's death, I think, was to see what my own could have been, had I not woken in that parking lot. I wanted to pay my respects, but whatever was once her body was caught up in the roots of a cypress. Death erases every bit of us, renders us anonymous. What remained of Lena was DNA, the final and most graceful human legacy. What a mystery that a human slipped out of her five months before she slipped to the floor. The mutated gene that I believe she carried—that I think her mother carried, that slept for a hundred years through generations of men—carved my story the way rushing rainwater sculpts a stream. I stood in the creek. I looked up at the banks, beyond the fences, to the flat area where the new owner raises quarter horses and hay. And then I gave up my search; I turned for town.

On the day of the surgery, the front-desk assistant at the cardiac catheterization lab sat me down in a small chair. "You are a car," she told me. "We open the hood. We take out the battery. We put in a new battery. We close the hood."

I looked at her squarely. "I. Am. A. Human," I said, and she rolled her eyes just enough for me to see it. "Cars don't get sepsis."

"You'll be fine," she said.

But I had been, in the past, a person for whom things were not fine, and so in the weeks leading up to surgery, my life twisted before me. The contract work I was paid for became impossible, unimportant. I found myself up late writing, or spending hours pushing myself on the trail. Here five miles. Here seven. Here nine, feeling my quads strengthen and tan, racing up hills under the desert sun. I went for forty-mile bike rides. I flew to Chicago to meet a man I'd been falling in love with from a distance, and we made out on every bridge downtown, ducking into alleyways to kiss against brick walls, riding the elevated train hand in hand. In the end, he closed our time together early, and I went home crushed, but I had known that this was part of living, and I wanted it. In the same way my body knew to have the surgery, it told me that something was coming. That I should drink these things down. That the way I lived now would matter.

My mom and I waited in the cardiac cath lab for hours, watching bad TV as my stomach growled. She had flown in the night before, on her sixty-first birthday, and I'd whisked her from the airport to a surprise party full of my friends—the last thing she expected on surgery duty. It had been a hard year. After Christine's device replacement in November, my dad had been diagnosed in December with prostate cancer. Although the procedure to remove his prostate in February had been successful and the cancer had not spread, my mom spent her winter sitting beside him in the hospital and at home as he suffered repeated bowel obstructions in the wake of the surgery, in agonizing pain and largely unable to eat. She'd long ago run out of paid time off from her job as a preschool teacher. When Melisa and I had landed in Chicago on our way to Colombia seven weeks before— laying over for the night at my parents'—my mom, no doubt hoping our visit would bring fresh energy into the house, had cheerfully and innocently asked, "How was your flight?"

I could only respond, "You're not going to believe this."

That night, the defibrillator's second set of warning vibrations woke me in the middle of the night in my childhood bedroom. Lying there among the familiar furniture, with the tops of the dark trees framed by the window, I wondered if things would be different if I were partnered—if the surgery would still fall so squarely on my parents. I wasn't twenty-four anymore. I had insurance. A wild sort of grief was opening up in me, something full of gratitude and fear at once. I had by then been single for nearly six years, and I knew what it meant to be immobilized, powerless, to have no choice but to lean on other humans. It scared me that at thirty, I was still leaning so hard on my mother.

I went out begging. "I need the defibrillator," I told them as the techs raised the blue paper surgical tent around me. "You have to give it to me. I've been writing a book about it for three and a half years. I've been all over the world researching it." The nurse, painting my chest with orange smears of antibiotic, shook her head. It was classified as a biohazard, she said. The hospital had to dispose of it.

"A man went home with his and later threw it in the trash," my St. Jude Medical technician, Jack, said. "The waste treatment facility found it, and St. Jude had to pay a big fine for improper disposal. So the policy changed."

"This will never show up in the trash," I pleaded.

Then, coming fuzzily awake. People telling me something important. Squinting, trying to focus. An X-ray clipped to the wall in front of me. The lead wire, one strip of it whiter and thinner than the rest. *The test failed. Clavicular crush.* The world in slow collapse as I understood: what was freshly stitched inside me was broken.

One of the nurses pushed a plastic lump into my hand. "Hide this," she hissed, walking away. It was a biohazard bag with a metal disk inside.

"I'll just dispose of this myself," the St. Jude rep said lightly, to no one in particular. "We can do it through the company just as easily." Gratitude pulsed through me. I clenched it hard beneath the blankets, this piece of me no longer me, this thing that lived inside my body for six and a half years, plugged into my heart. It was what I had to hold on to as I learned what was next. Like the ashes of a lover I would carry it home.

At the quiet end of surgery, as the encore of every defibrillator placement, there is a test: the surgical team induces an arrhythmia and waits for the ICD to correct it. I imagine this moment, the surgeon's eyes flickering up across my body to lock with the St. Jude rep's after the shock rolled in and the heart did not stop quivering.

A lead wire is a metal coil slipped into a polyurethane-silicon sleeve and laced down the veins all the way to the heart. On the tip of the lead wire is a corkscrew with a steroid up its middle to stimulate scar-tissue growth. Once the lead wire is in place—gently twisted into the wall of the ventricle or atrium—it must stay in place, sensing rhythm and delivering electricity accurately. The lead wire is in it for the long haul, plugged into the header of one defibrillator after another.

Or ideally it will be.

In the X-ray the cath lab team pinned above my bed, the wire went strangely flat, crushed between my clavicle and first rib, the rest of it continuing in an elegant, thin rope toward the tricuspid valve. The crack had likely happened years ago, they told me, but the coating on the wire had been held in place by the scar tissue around it. Only when they jostled the wire while pulling the old ICD out and plugging the new ICD in did the insulation move enough to be detected, to actually fail.

Was I at risk all those months, when my old ICD was testing normally in medical offices? We'd never know. But the new ICD inside me might not work at all; when the voltage didn't correctly make it to the heart during the test, it could have discharged into the device itself, frying the ICD's circuitry in some hard-to-detect way. They'd need to open me up, either to attempt to remove the broken wire, or to tie it off forever. In the process, they'd remove my potentially ruined second ICD and lace a new wire down my veins. Abruptly, I would be on to my third defibrillator.

By the time I learned lead wires could fail, I'd had my own for two and a half years. In the late spring of 2012, my dad forwarded

Christine and me a *New York Times* article titled "Device Malfunction Casts Doubt on Industry Pledge," about the St. Jude Medical Riata lead wire. The Riata had been recalled that December after twenty patient deaths—eerily referred to as "high-voltage fatalities" by one physician—revealed a pattern of insulation abrasion, in which internal cables rubbed their way through their coatings.

What wires do you ladies have? Dad wrote.

I don't know, but that is creepy.

I think you need to find out. I think you have St. Jude, he said.

In the article, *Times* reporters Barry Meier and Katie Thomas tell the story of a cardiac device industry with a history not only of FDA recalls but also of negligent responses to the first inklings of trouble with devices and their components. In 2002, defibrillator maker Guidant (now part of Boston Scientific) failed to warn doctors about a flaw that was causing some defibrillators to short-circuit. The company ultimately pleaded guilty to two misdemeanors, paid $296 million, and accepted three years of probation for having hidden the defects for more than three years. In 2007 Medtronic recalled its Sprint Fidelis lead wire after its coating began cracking inside patients, amid widespread scrutiny about when and how much it had known about dangers to patients. As the cardiac-device historian Kirk Jeffrey notes in his book *Machines in Our Hearts,* whereas "early deaths were, in a sense, part of the price society paid for the growth of knowledge about artificially managing the heartbeat and implanting electronic devices within the human body," product failures in interventions that have "gained acceptance as . . . normal procedure[s] . . . [receive] a much higher level of unsympathetic public attention."

Unwind a paper clip in your hands and wiggle it back and forth, back and forth, to see how long before the metal snaps. In *Machines in Our Hearts,* Jeffrey writes about the lead wire as a feat of engineering, for the heart is a muscle of constant movement, and the sensing of rhythm—the delivery of electricity—a precise art. "At 70 contractions per minute, the heart beats 36,792,000 times in a year," Jeffrey notes. A lead wire must not only withstand the pressures of the body—the heart's constant flexing, the valve flapping open and shut, a general dampness, the sensitivity of tissue and blood to foreign objects, the tendency for tissue to grow on a foreign body in the heart—but also discern rhythms and conduct electricity reliably.

The earliest wires to transmit electricity to the human heart were designed for pacemakers, not ICDs. Pacemakers at their invention were not the matchbox-size devices we know today but hulking machinery on carts, plugged into the wall, with external electrodes placed against the chest. Initially, pacemakers were invented to resuscitate and keep alive patients with partial or complete heart block, a condition in which the ventricles don't receive electrical messages from the atrium and thus beat poorly. "Because the electrodes were not in direct contact with heart tissue, a stimulus of 30 to 150 volts was required to drive the ventricles," writes Jeffrey. "This caused involuntary contraction of chest muscles and, for most patients, proved too painful for extended use."

"Getting a shock like that fifty, sixty times a minute is torture," said Dr. C. Walton Lillehei, who performed some of the first open heart surgeries to repair ventricular septal defects in young children. His young patients would occasionally develop heart block after the procedures—a sign that his stitching had interfered with the heart's electrical conductivity—and external pacemakers often kept them alive for several weeks while their hearts' conduction systems healed. "With some of the infants, we were able to restrain them so they wouldn't tear [the chest electrodes] off, but they would develop blisters and ulcers [beneath the electrodes] in four to five days. So that was totally inadequate." Another cardiac innovator, Seymour Furman, told the story of a patient who had been on one of the original external pacemakers for "a long time" and "finally committed suicide by turning off the switch just after a pep talk which the house staff, myself included, had given him about the wonders of the future to come, which we didn't believe and he equally didn't believe."

The next generation of pacemakers were boxes worn around the neck, with a light that flashed each time electricity stimulated the heart. The wires ran through an open port in the patients' chests, which left an easy route to infection and proved hard for patients to ignore; however, the placement of the wires directly on the heart enabled pacing with a lower (and more humane) voltage. The earliest pacemaker wires broke regularly, an emergency for patients who relied on the device for their every heartbeat, and—in these years before pacemakers were implanted transvenously—required that the chest be opened back up. Early pacemaker engineers worried that the constantly flexing wires would dig a hole in the myocardium and fussed over the different types of electrodes that would adorn their tips, noting the way the "movement, stressing, and flexing…could likely irritate tissue and cause the fibrotic buildup to become larger." If this buildup occurred, it would take larger amounts of electricity to maintain continuous pacing, running down the battery of the device more quickly.

While a number of teams of physicians and engineers experimented with different metals and methods of soldering the electrode, seeking consistency and longevity, it was the pacemaker engineer William Chardack who, in 1961, came across a promising orthodontic spring, able to flex for long periods without breaking. He adapted it for use in the heart. The first coiled-spring myocardial lead was a mixture of platinum and iridium and quickly established itself as "the first reliable pacemaker lead." It was, as Jeffrey writes, "the starting-point for later lead designs"—including lead wires for the ICD.

The first ICD was implanted in a human in 1980, approved by the FDA for public release in 1985, and accepted as a reimbursable procedure by Medicare in 1986. Bulky and implanted in the abdomen, these early devices' lead wires attached to the heart through an incision in the chest wall. By 1988, the ICD, like the pacemaker, had moved to transvenous leads—implanted in a cardiac catheterization lab instead of through open chest surgery. Over time the industry transitioned from a coaxial lead—in which the tip conductor, ring conductor, and defibrillation conductor nested like matryoshka dolls, with a layer of insulation between each conductor—to a multilumen lead, which allowed parallel conductors to run through a single insulating body, with additional open channels present "to increase the lead's resistance to compression forces," according to a 2011 article published in the *Netherlands Heart Journal*.

The most common industrywide source of lead failure, though, remained the insulation of the wire, which protects the interior conductors from the juices, movements, and inconsistencies of the body. The first lead wires were insulated with silicone rubber (a technology borrowed from roller pumps), which was adequately bio-stable and flexible but was susceptible to abrasion, both from without and from within. By the late 1970s, manufacturers were borrow-ing technology used in undersea telephone cables, insulating wires with polyurethane 80A—which proved to have poor biostability—and polyurethane 55D, which proved to be too stiff.

And so the 2011 failure and recall of the St. Jude Medical Riata wire was only the latest of its type, arriving into public light after several years in which the company—and its board of independent specialists—quietly monitored the problem, years during which critics say the company should have been alerting cardiologists. Once they did send out the letter of caution, the FDA quickly forced a Class I recall. "In a recent study at Vanderbilt," write Meier and Thomas, "researchers found that about a third of Riata leads in patients they examined showed signs of protruding wires. Nearly a third of those showed electrical failures."

As it turned out, I didn't have the Riata wire. By luck, my ICD and wires were implanted just after St. Jude released the Durata. The Durata, St. Jude's engineers told me when I called, was coated by their new insulator Optim—an abrasion-resistant polyurethane-silicon polymer that formed a protective jacket around the lead—and thus had nothing to do with the recall. I was relieved. Medtronic had, by then, added a similar protective sheath to their next-generation Sprint Quattro lead. Still, a 2015 study published in the *Journal of the American Heart Association* by Rui Providencia, et al., suggests that—while differences in lead failure rates among models built by all three major manufacturers could be attributed to lead design elements—the rates of failure themselves were "non-negligible" for all models.

Lead wires fail at rates that matter, no matter who manufac-tures them.

All this engineering, all these ways to fail. Yet having only heard of lead failure related to mass defects, I was caught off guard by my own wire's deterioration. It was so simple: the wire had gotten crunched. In the murmurings after I woke up, someone said the wire may have been placed too high, someone said the wire may have migrated too high over time. At five foot three, I am a small human, and even though the wires came in sixty-, sixty-five-, and seventy-five-centimeter lengths, it's possible I ended up with more centimeters than I should have, driving a high loop between the header of the generator and the heart. Later, after I researched, I wouldn't know whether to blame the Durata's lead design for not absorbing enough compression when the wire slipped into that space between my first rib and clavicle, or whether to blame myself—whether my arm rising up for a climbing hold or a sun salutation was the source of the pinch, a risk I hadn't known was there. The technology, as always, matched best the sedentary lives of the elderly.

But that afternoon, sitting up in bed in the cardiac catheterization recovery room, I had almost no context for what had happened. My surgeon never arrived to explain. It was the St. Jude Medical rep, smiling kindly, who popped in at my bedside to see how I was, to begin explaining the decisions that lay before me.

And so the recovery was a false one. For two days my mother and I sat in a rented casita at the edge of the desert and watched the Gambel's quail and Gila woodpeckers peck at the ground outside the door, clouds sending long shadows across the yellowing golf courses and swooped mountains. Once again, my mother helped me kneel in the bathtub, running a washcloth over my body while I held a towel and plastic bag over my sutures.

There was so much less pain than I expected, and my body, strong and vital, hitched the two sides of the incision together without complaint. But all that time I knew the incision would be reopened shortly, and this gave the whole weekend an air of unreality. In truth I could feel once more the slow collapse of my horizon, the way a month of plans and obligations shift and shatter, the way the self empties in the face of illness. A surgery or health crisis requires of us a radical, forced form of presence: for a time, there can be only *this*.

For the removal of a wire grown into the heart would be no

small thing, I learned in the days after they discovered the fracture. In this instance a doctor would slide a long straw, known as a laser sheath, over the lead wire, following it down my vein all the way into my ventricle. Lasers on the end of the straw—similar to those used in LASIK procedures, which dissolve fibrous tissue into microscopic shreds that can be absorbed by the bloodstream—would cut the wire from the heart.

Like all advanced technology, this sounded so precise, so well controlled; in some instances it is. Yet one afternoon I began to read white papers online that made it real. For a human being, even if enhanced with metal and polyurethane, is made of tissue, is shreddable. The superior vena cava—the big vein delivering blood to the heart— can be nicked by the edges of the laser sheath. Scar tissue can clench the lead with a ferocity we don't expect. The myocardium, the layer of heart muscle that received the wire so many years ago, can easily rip. If it bleeds into the space beside the pericardium—the outer muscle of the heart—the heart can't pump, a condition called cardiac tamponade. For this reason surgery would be performed not in the cardiac catheterization lab, like my other procedures, but in a hybrid facility also used for open heart surgery, with a team standing by ready to carve open my sternum to stanch the bleeding. Major complication rates for the procedure hovered between 1 and 2 percent, and the mortality rate was not negligible. One should have the procedure only in a major surgery center, I read, where individual surgeons perform these delicate motions more than a hundred times a year.

I found myself placing my fingers against my breastbone, so soft and unsevered. I touched my skin and just breathed.

The other option, of course, was to just leave the cracked wire in place. They could tie it off—there were people who had three of these, five of these, seven of these, all still corkscrewed into the heart, a graveyard of leads. My own tailings field. Here, again, the questions were different for a person who was young, who would be accruing lead wires, if she were lucky, for another fifty years. In the same way the idea of getting an ICD immediately nauseated me, the idea of carrying detritus panicked me. The problem was this: if a person's heart becomes infected, all leads need to be immediately removed or the infection cannot be excised from the body. The metal becomes a fort for bacteria. This was why Dr. Oza had ordered those pictures of my heart, taken down my throat, when I was septic; whether the infection was on my lead wires dictated whether the lead wires got to stay.

The problem of sepsis is common among those who are aging, often part of a cascade of events that send a person's health tumbling. In those instances, even with the wires removed, people might die; there's so much going on that the risk of the procedure is, if not negligible, at least only one determining factor among many. But I'd been a twenty-four-year-old who began rotting alive. At thirty, I was not so stupid as to think myself immune. To hear the word *sepsis* made me go shaky inside. The role the wires played would be decisive.

It was true as well that wires became more difficult to remove over time. Which meant that the wire would never be easier to remove than it was at that moment. If I waited until later, and it could not be removed—if this happened while I was septic again—what then?

At my follow-up appointment, I finally saw Dr. Garrick for the first time since the preoperation appointment where we'd met. He was a lean, blond-haired man who always looked vaguely like he'd just leaped off a treadmill. In the cath lab, the techs and nurses had marveled aloud at his reputation as a surgeon, his ability to leave a slender scar line devoid of keloid. I tried to tell myself that this was what mattered, but I knew, too, that after what I'd been through—and with what I was facing—I needed a doctor who could be in conversation not just with my technical mind, but also with my fear and intuition.

That day Dr. Garrick assured me that there was no reason we had to make an immediate decision on extracting the lead, that it could be capped off and left indefinitely. The main decision at hand, he said, was whether or not to replace the ICD before I went abroad, knowing that what was inside me might be fried, might not work as intended. And if we replaced the ICD before I went, we'd have to implant a new, functional wire. Attempting an extraction of the old wire later, then, might jostle or upset the new wire in some way, but this didn't mean we couldn't put the extraction off at this point if I wasn't ready.

It was a Wednesday. He could get me on the schedule for a wire removal, if I wanted, for a week from that day, on May 11. I told him I had read procedures of this type should only be performed in major surgery centers; the community hospital where he had admitting privileges was not one of these. He reassured me: if I booked the surgery, there was someone who traveled the Rocky Mountain region performing just these procedures at smaller hospitals who would be called in.

There was another option, though, Dr. Garrick said. A new type of ICD was gaining traction, and I might be a good candidate for it. The subcutaneous ICD (S-ICD) was implanted beneath the skin but above the ribs, he told me, so that there were no wires actually in your veins, which removed much of the risk of the transvenous ICDs we were used to. About the size of a makeup compact or a thick wallet, the S-ICD was an oblong brick placed beneath the armpit, with its wires tunneled along the ribs and into the space between the breasts, where an electrode near—but not in—the heart sensed and shocked. The invention was akin to a half step between the ICD I'd carried for the previous six and a half years, and external defibrillators like the paddles in the ER, the AEDs that hang on the walls of airports, and the wearable defibrillator called the LifeVest that sometimes serves as a bridge to surgery (with its bra straps and built-in dry conductors that shoot gel against your skin before they shock you).

Dr. Garrick's enthusiasm for the S-ICD caught me a little off guard; I'd never heard of the thing, and now he seemed to be pushing for it. I went home and read. First approved by the FDA in 2012, the S-ICD in 2016 seemed still to be getting on its feet, though its concept proved to be a game changer for those who didn't need to be paced, for the young who were suffering the side effects of wires accumulating in their veins. But the device was still big and blocky, more than twice the size of my current ICD—a result of the increased voltage and generating capacity required to shock the heart from the outside. It also seemed the S-ICD's sensing might not be dialed in yet—I read about higher rates of accidental shocks.

In an attempt to understand the device beyond the glossy Boston Scientific advertisements that filled the internet, I joined an S-ICD

Facebook group, posting questions about yoga and climbing, asking if there were any young women who would be willing to share pictures of what the device really looked like against their bodies. The women I messaged with were enthusiastic, so grateful to have the wires gone from their veins, so grateful to have this other option for saving their lives. Yes, they did yoga: no problem.

Then the pictures rolled in: grotesque bulges atop ribs. Red scar lines hanging to the curve of breasts. The slit at the sternum where the wires ended. Unnatural bumps on the side of the female body that made my stomach turn forcefully, not unlike what would happen if I saw a leg broken at a dramatic angle.

I stood in the mirror, shirtless, turning and looking. Touching my beautiful rib cage. The smooth skin hugging it. Imagining the way that spot felt to a man, his palm against the curve of me. I pictured my body on the climbing wall, mantling, what it would mean if the side that scraped the wall had an enormous electronic bulge. I was thirty. I could hardly look at the pictures. I knew my younger sister had at some points been self-conscious about the bulge in her chest. But for me the rise of it had been so slight, easily hidden in my breast tissue. *This* would lump out of every shirt I owned.

I must love my own beauty too much, I wrote in my journal.

"I must not be dying enough," I told my friends.

In the gleam in Dr. Garrick's eye I had seen an excitement, a desire to be part of the latest technology, and something about that filled me with rage. As though I were a lab rat, I found myself thinking. I asked myself if my response would be different if the technology were older, if the pulse generator were smaller and the shocks more precise, if I was less likely to be part of a test cohort, the "early adopters." I understood that a device could be optimistically released to the public and still be in development for a long while. A technology is worth it, as pacemaker innovator Dwight Harken had said, "when its use is safer for the patient than the prognosis of his disease, and is the best available." I didn't know if the S-ICD was the best treatment available. And as each year passed without cardiac arrest—my ICD silent despite my lack of beta-blockers, my device checks noting no unusual rhythms—I didn't know if the technology was safer than the prognosis of my disease. What, actually, did long QT mean for me? What did a transvenous ICD mean versus a subcutaneous one?

The decision makes for a bad essay, I wrote in my journal. *It is not necessarily rational. It is bodily. My body says no.*

Now the heat of the summer came to Tucson, the flare of sun that would cook the desert brown. I walked up and down the block, gathering strength. I read academic paper after academic paper. It turned out all roads lead to death. I could avoid the risk of the procedure by not having it, but then I would have to live with the question of whether to put a second wire into the heart beside the abandoned first. Or I could avoid the risks of all this imperfect technology by simply opting out—by leaving quiet the broken lead in my heart, by having the potentially broken defibrillator in my chest turned off and abandoned. By finally calling it, and giving in to the risks of long QT.

The death I felt courting me then, at nearly thirty-one, was gentler and quieter than the death I had come to know at twenty-four. It felt like a language I had come to speak: if not an old friend, then at least a presence I understood how to dance with. My body was only the size that it was, small in the world. I could die on the operating table or in a parking lot, I realized, circling the block. I could die crossing the street in Tucson or in a traffic accident in some African city, or I could die in sixty years, striped from the incisions of new defibrillators, my skin ratty from fluoroscopy, my endocardium pebbled with scar tissue from parades of lead wires. I was afraid, but I was not as afraid as I used to be.

All things were dangerous, which meant none of them were.

I would do the lead extraction now, while I was young and strong. And I would take a new ICD inside me to Tanzania for my job.

Two nights before my lead extraction surgery I went for a walk that was intended to be a block but turned into a mile, wandering the wide gravel streets as the darkness came down. I pressed my face into the night blooms of the oleander, sharp white in the dim light. The air was silk. Down near the elementary school, I sighted a lump along the telephone wire, something quavery that at first looked like a cat preening, but so high off the ground.

Once I was underneath it, I knew: an owl. I circled from all sides, trying to be sure, startled that it hadn't flown off. Then I sat before it for a long time, watching a bright fingernail of moon go down behind it. The twin pyramids of ears were visible in that light: it was a great horned.

An owl sighting means death, this much I remembered, although from where I could not say. Owls visit those who are dying, but not in the physical sense; death, in the spiritual realm, always means this sloughing, change that comes with force, the way a life turns over into something else. Owls draw attention to timing. Owls have the particular gift of seeing in the dark, of using the tiny bit of light that is there.

On the sidewalk before the owl, I said aloud, "Let me see your eyes."

Minutes of silence, the neighborhood deep blue, the stars arriving overhead. Then one car swung toward us from the south, headlights bright, wheels skidding over some gravel on the road. The owl, at the last minute, swiveled her face. After so much murkiness: hot orange eyes, powerful and terrible, trained on me. The owl swept off the wire, landed on the ground ten feet before me, then rose back to the telephone wire. And when I finally went, I could not turn away from her; I walked backward down the block, eyes fastened on her as long as I could keep them, and she lifted off the wire just as I turned the corner, a giant dark wingspan pivoting away.

If illness forces us to be present—the threat of death bringing us abruptly, even nonconsensually, into the moment—I was grateful for it then. I touched my wet face and breathed in the smell of the desert. Forget the wreckage of the calendar and the bank account this month of surgeries had wrought. I was alive.

My mother flew back to town, sleeping on the futon in my living room. We drove to the surgery center first thing in the morning, my belly empty with the required fasting. I tried to train my eyes on every single building I passed on Grant Road. These could be the last things I saw alive. The day was already hot. I had not in a long time prayed, but I did as I put on my hospital gown, as I emptied my earrings into the plastic hospital bag, as I slipped out my nose ring. A nurse arrived to shave my pubic hair. "Oh," I said. "I must have missed the memo on this appointment." She smiled grimly but did not seem to think her task was as funny as I found it. I was a woman who proudly never so much as trimmed her pubic area, now recipient of her first nonconsensual shave.

"For a femoral incision," she said, "it's a matter of creating a sterile environment."

"I didn't know I was getting a femoral incision," I told her.

"You're not, necessarily," she said. But in case anything changed, the surgeon needed it to be prepped and sterile.

"Huh," I said.

Later, I would wish I were paying closer attention in the surgery center, to the sequence of people coming in and out. I met the anesthesiologist. Dr. Garrick ducked in to say hello, and when I asked where the person was who toured the whole Rocky Mountain region performing this procedure, he looked sideways at me. "Oh, the Cook Medical rep," he said. "We weren't able to get him at the last minute." *A medical rep? Is that the guy I thought was coming? I thought it was a practitioner, who only does this procedure?* Just as my mind was beginning to work on the problem—*Wait, is it just Dr. Garrick, then? But all the studies said—should I be going into this surgery?*—the anesthesia was flowing, the bed was rolling, I said goodbye to my mother and was gone.

To wake from a surgery can mean waking into a nightmare. The nurse stood over me, angry. The edges of everything fuzzy. "This will hurt," she said darkly. "They're supposed to do this while you're still under." Then her mouth filled with words I could not understand: *The procedure failed. The wire broke off.* All at once she pulled the sheath from my femoral incision and slammed the heel of her hand into my groin, and I was screaming. "Stop that," she said harshly. "We have to get a clot to form or you'll bleed in spurts every time your heart beats, because in the femoral the pressure is high, coming right from the heart." But I was not in control of the sounds of me, so sharp red the sensation, the most painful moment of my life. She slid a slender metal arm over the side of the bed and cranked a black knob as the pain in my groin exploded, and I saw it was a C-clamp, not unlike the kind I'd used in industrial arts class in sixth grade to hold wood while I sawed along a carefully penciled line. Now I was clamped to the bed by my groin, in the fold where my right thigh began. "Twenty minutes," she said, and I tried to breathe, tried to follow my breath out of screaming, but none of the lines of the room were right, there was only that jagged red pain.

Later she would release the clamp and look at me fiercely. "Now you cannot move for six hours, do you understand?" I was not to sit up in the slightest, because it could cause a rush of blood to the groin and dislodge the tender clot we'd built, and then we'd be back where we had started. I was not to laugh or sneeze or cough. If I felt something coming I could push my hand where the incision had been, to hold the clot in place.

Then into a cramped, shabby room, where a woman who'd just come out of open heart surgery moaned and snored on the other side of the curtain, her monitors beeping. The new nurse—a more compact, cheerier woman—began to attach the automatic blood pressure cuff to my left arm. "No," I said. "I have a fresh incision on that side." I needed to be able to keep my arm at a protective angle. But in my right arm ran all the IV lines, bruises already pooling inside my elbow and forearm. With my right leg off-limits because of the femoral incision, the blood pressure cuff went on my left calf, the muscles getting painfully squeezed each hour through the night.

As the anesthesia ebbed, in rushed the nausea I'd heard about, a horrible lurching, a cheek-flushing sourness. "We can give you something for that," the nurse said.

"Excuse me," I said, "I just want to make sure you saw that I'm a long QT patient. If it's what I think it is, it's on my drugs-to-avoid list. Please be sure you check my contraindications."

"Oh, no, it should be fine," the nurse said.

"I need you to double-check," I said. "When I've come out of anesthesia in the past, I haven't been allowed anything."

"Well, you have an ICD," the nurse said. "That's what it's for!"

She wasn't joking.

Mom and I exchanged horrified looks. "You're going to give me a drug that could put me in cardiac arrest because it's fine, I have a *de-fibrillator*? Which would go off under my fresh incision? At a moment I'm not supposed to move at all because I could dislodge a femoral clot? Are you crazy?" I said.

At that moment, my mom and I knew she wouldn't be leaving that night. She would sleep sitting up in a chair, if she slept at all. The care I was receiving felt scary. If something happened in the wake of the surgery and I couldn't advocate for myself, someone else would need to be there, not several miles away; the nurse's judgment couldn't be trusted. I thought of the eyes of the owl. It was easy to think that once my six hours lying flat were up, the medical part of my stay would be over, but someone had been tugging at the thinnest part of my heart, sticking technical tools up my veins and arteries. If there was a slow bleed, we might not know about it right away. If there was a clot. Here began a long night.

For the first time, I understood what it meant to have only a single insurer on the health-care marketplace, as was the case in Pima County. Though it had looked like I had options as I perused the government website—though I had been gleeful about getting insurance at all—those options had to do with the math of copays, deductibles, and premiums, not networks. In that realm, I'd had no choice: there was one insurer. My surgery would be at this community hospital. I could choose between Dr. Garrick and one other electro-physiologist at another office, the only practitioners in town willing to accept low negotiated rates in return for the influx of new patients the market provided. And having lived in wealthy communities such as Boulder and Jackson, where the health-care facilities invariably met a certain standard, it hadn't occurred to me that a community hospital could be inadequate. Everyone at this hospital, I tried to reassure myself, had the appropriate medical licenses; the surgery center where I'd begun my day was state-of-the-art, bright and new, a recent renovation. I tried to be fair, to differentiate between flashy and adequate. Even at nice facilities, I'd struggled to get practitioners to listen to me. But I'd assumed, by and large, that if I could get them to listen to my symptoms, they'd catch the patterns. They'd have an answer. That night, however, it felt like something important would be missed. Tucson was a scrappy place, a city of half a million that felt rural in so many ways. One of my dearest friends, Janelle, worked in the cardiac ICU over at University Medical Center, and I knew it was the magnet for regional heart patients, the only hospital of its caliber in our area, offering advanced technologies, the most capable surgeons, and nurses who tend to people like me regularly. A care team will be good at whatever it practices regularly. In a place like Tucson, it mattered which hospital I used for a relatively rare high-risk procedure—and so it made all the difference where my insurance would allow me to go.

I followed my breath in the most careful sips, my body spinning with nausea.

A mouth, denied water for a whole day, dries and aches. Late at night my mother fed me one ice chip at a time with a plastic spoon, angling them into my mouth while I lay absolutely flat, patient and careful. Officially, I wasn't supposed to have anything until the six hours were up, because vomiting carried the risk of either dislodging my femoral clot or causing me to aspirate. I could see how very tired my mother was. How she was getting older. It had been late afternoon when I woke out of surgery. Now it was lurching toward 10:00 p.m., and we knew the cafeteria would be limited at this hour and generally dismal. I asked her to send a text to several of my friends, pleading for the delivery of a vanilla milkshake. My mom laughed. "You and your milkshakes," she said. When I was septic, it had been one of the only things I'd eaten well—a bourbon vanilla milkshake from one of the bars downtown. My mother had wandered in, skeptical, wearing her raincoat. "Do you guys have...milkshakes?" she said, eyeing the tall wall of liquor bottles, expecting them to laugh. But they didn't laugh, and they did have milkshakes, and she took the Styrofoam cup of thick liquid back to the third floor of Boulder Community Hospital and slipped the straw into my mouth. Now, with an hour until midnight, finally allowed to minimally move, my dear friends Kat and Alison arrived into that dark, horrible hospital room and brought us laughter, a moment's break, my mom carefully spooning the milkshake into my mouth. This, I had learned, was what love looked like at the edge of all things: people who could bear to be with you in pain without looking away, and who did whatever small thing they could to ease it.

Picture the moment:

After they fixed the top of the wire with thread in the defibrillator pocket, after they tried to inch the laser sheath down the wire, the lead snapped and fell away down the vein. The surgical team moved to the femoral artery, an attempt to capture it from below. The surgeon placed a sheath more than five millimeters in diameter and extended a Needle's Eye Snare—like a tiny shepherd's crook made of wire—upward through it, into the inferior vena cava, to capture the broken lead. *Got it.* He pulled it into the sheath, his movements careful, and advanced the sheath until he was within two centimeters of the lead tip. Then pulled.

On the fluoroscopy screen, the whole heart lurched. My systolic blood pressure plummeted to 40. The surgeon released the traction; my blood pressure recovered. He twisted the sheath, hoping, tugging as much as felt safe. Any more, he knew, and the heart could tear.

In the operative report, the paragraph ends quietly: "The lead was abandoned."

In the morning the attending physician would ask what I was there for, and I would have to explain my presence, only narrowly holding back my anger, full of sharp things I might say to suggest that she could have looked at my chart before she walked into the room. Her eyes widened as she heard what had happened. I resented being an interesting case; I was, through my insurance, paying her for this worthless stop she made in my room, where I entertained her, offered my life as gossip and anecdote. What I could tell her about what happened I was cobbling together from what the nurse had said during my sheath removal and what my mom told me; Dr. Garrick had at least found my mother in the waiting room after the procedure to fill her in. But he had never come to see me—a thirty-year-old woman who made her own health-care decisions, whose brain was by nature more technical than her mother's, who had her own questions and fears. He never reappeared to explain what had happened—to in some small way hand me back my future.

When I went to see him the next week at his practice, I would be told I was actually seeing his physician's assistant, and my voice would rise in panic and rage. His office assistants angled their heads conspiratorially, suggesting that the PA made up for what the surgeon lacked when it came to talking to patients. And indeed, the PA was some comfort, wearing green scrubs, with curly dark hair and a kind face, making eye contact. He had at least been in the room when it happened. He could tell me how on the fluoroscopy they saw my vascular system lift. But it was not the same as being looked in the eye by the man under whose hand the wire had snapped, the man who had pulled hard on debris stuck in my heart.

Once I had my medical records, I would understand that Dr. Garrick had come to an edge where he might have pulled harder, where he could have been stubborn, hubristic—and he had not. He had not ripped my heart; I had not woken with a cleaved sternum, or died. He had stepped humbly back. The lead was abandoned. I respected him for this. And yet what I wanted was not an apology, exactly, but the kind of "I'm sorry" that acknowledged what this would mean in my life. It was a form of accountability to stand with one's patients no matter the outcome. To really see the outcome—which, I knew, changed the way one worked with other patients. It changed the way one weighed the use of medical technologies.

Accountability required vulnerability; it was therefore something hard, not necessarily fun. It required prioritizing showing up. "A core social expectation of being sick is surrendering oneself to the care of a physician," writes socionarratologist Arthur Frank. "I understand this obligation of seeking medical care as a narrative surrender...[But] more is involved in [patients'] experiences than the medical story can tell. The loss of a life's map and destination are not medical symptoms."

If Dr. Garrick had gotten the wire out, he would have been a hero. The technological tools he used, too, would have seemed heroic. Never mind that—like the lauded conservation offset that accompanies a mine pit—this "heroism" merely sought to fix the previous failure. My rage was that of someone who had surrendered her narrative, of an unconscious body, the blank stage upon which the drama was performed. Without Dr. Garrick's presence, it didn't matter how many white papers I'd read: I could not access all the pieces of my own story. I could not know what had happened to my body. If there is a better definition of trauma than that, I cannot think of one. The procedure failed medically because the wire snapped— because it would remain there dangling in my vena cava into an unknown future. But the team failed narratively because they left me alone without the story of my body. I awoke into narrative wreckage. The physician's assistant who was supposed to console me was a stranger—and a week late.

That night after surgery, unmoored, I would manage my own care lying on my back, and ride the nausea and thrumming pain without really understanding what had happened. I would nearly cry out of relief when Jack the St. Jude Medical rep poked his head around the corner with his wheeled cart bearing ICD programmer and wand, which may as well have been a white horse. I would soften when he smiled at me, ready to tell me the story—the only professional passing through my room who was not employed by the hospital and yet the only one dressing the wound that most needed dressing—able to act like he cared.

If you had seen me in those weeks afterward, the scar would have looked good. The scar would have looked like lips pressed together, neat and calm, a mouth covering a new defibrillator plugged into a new wire, carefully angled into the right ventricle to avoid the old one, going about the careful work of growing into my heart. But what you would not see was the debris, the coil tip and electrode of the old wire buried firmly in the thinnest part of my heart, a dangerous place to yank. The wire was a white ghost in my veins, flapping in the weather of my body. And I could not stop thinking of a wet wind of blood, its rhythmic pouring. The way tissue colonizes everything like mold or moss in the dank northern cities. The possibility that the loose wire could cause "noise" in my new electrical circuit, even trigger shocks. How eventually the slack body of the wire might drift toward the inferior vena cava; how someday the metal of the wire could eat its way through the too-soft insulation, sending debris into circulation. I woke late one night in a panic when my hands—often tucked into the waistband of my underwear when I sleep as a sort of weighted comfort—fell upon a hard bulb in my inner thigh where the incision had been. With a hand mirror in the middle of the night I could see its bruising, old by then, the puff of its bandage recently pulled off and thrown away. I was convinced the knob was plastic shed by the wire, or a dangerous clot, and was reassured only in the morning by a dismissive on-call doctor: it was just my femoral clot. It would take a while to dissolve. I should push against it, but only gently.

I could see, then, the error of my thinking. The removal of the wire had become to me a do-over: something I thought I could undergo bravely to fix the problems of the technology, to clean up the mess. It was scary, but I could start fresh. If I cleaned up the mess of the technology, I could clean up death itself. I could stop thinking about it, declare it again distant and irrelevant. But the body is a story always advancing toward one end. A wire is just one reminder. And even when we recover from a condition, we never return to what we were; we become different, host to debris both spiritual and physical. Now the fear I carried of sepsis would be forever visceral. That noodle of a wire, oxbowing quietly down my vena cava, wasn't dangerous then. But it would be someday. None of us could say when.

CAUSA MATERIALIS

CHAPTER 13

Busoro, Rwanda
2016

The first mine I entered with a broken wire was a hand-dug shaft on the eastern shore of Lake Kivu, in western Rwanda—a sandy, cool tunnel barely wide enough to put one arm out sideways. Since the 1930s, men had followed this vein of wolframite, cassiterite, and coltan into the ground, but only recently had it been certified as "conflict free." That's what sent me south out of Gisenyi on a motorbike, clutching a man named Jonah as he steered up and down the hills toward the tiny town of Busoro. Across the water, everything was Congo until the Atlantic.

The night I took two thousand volts to the heart, the question that landed in my body was most distinctly about these minerals, in this part of the world. Wolframite: the source of tungsten, used to make a cell phone—or a defibrillator with a low battery—vibrate. Cassiterite: tin, used as a solder on circuit boards. Coltan: the local name for tantalum, a mineral critical for storing electricity in electronics, dug up in this region as columbite-tantalite. These, together with gold, were the famed conflict minerals, mined by hand in pits controlled by armed groups across the border in the Democratic Republic of the Congo, smuggled into legitimate markets in Rwanda and Uganda, and sold on the global market at high prices driven by the demand for consumer electronics such as laptops and smartphones.

In 2012, the year I was shocked, headlines on social media

proclaimed the DRC the "rape capital of the world," referring to the armed groups that had proliferated in the region after Rwanda's 1994 genocide and the First and Second Congo Wars that followed. I was the kind of person who clicked through, who read about the traumatic fistulas suffered by women unlucky enough to be caught in the way: vaginal tissues torn so severely that a hole opened between the vagina and rectum or bladder, creating leaks and infections. I read about the women kept as sex slaves, the young boys seeking opportunity who found their way to the pits and slid underground, into hot tunnels wet with shit and piss, to hammer veins of tin—only to find they'd incurred too much "debt" by their presence to ever leave.

Some of the armed groups were Mai-Mai: local militias originally sprung up to protect villages during war, many of which then turned to the same raping, pillaging, and child soldier–conscripting tactics they'd suffered. Some were defectors from the Congolese army who rebelled against the government of President Joseph Kabila. And although Rwanda and Uganda officially withdrew their troops from the DRC by 2002, each backed rebel factions there, fighting a proxy war. In 2017, the Africa Center for Strategic Studies estimated that at least seventy armed groups were operating in the DRC, the vast majority of them located in the eastern provinces—North Kivu, South Kivu, and Ituri—and numbering fewer than two hundred troops each.

One thing was clear: every armed group had figured out how to get paid when their faraway governments or warlord leaders failed to provide. The Congo has been referred to as "a geological scandal," and with mineral prices soaring, controlling mines was lucrative.

In July of 2010, the United States passed the Dodd-Frank Act, financial reform legislation crafted in response to the 2008 global financial crisis. The legislation included an unrelated rider known as the "conflict minerals provision," the result of years of lobbying by nongovernmental organizations who'd been investigating the ongoing violence in the DRC. The rider, Section 1502, required companies listed on U.S. stock exchanges to file an annual report publicly disclosing whether their products contain any tin, tantalum, tungsten, or gold—known as 3TG—"necessary to [the product's] functionality or production" and whether these minerals originated in the Democratic

Republic of the Congo "or an adjoining country." If the minerals did come from one of these nations, the company was then required to follow a "due diligence" process to identify the minerals' "chain of custody," including their original source, and to learn whether they may have financed or benefited armed groups. The regulation, I knew, roughly followed the model of the Kimberley Process, a program initiated by the United Nations General Assembly in response to the diamond-fueled wars in Sierra Leone, Liberia, and Angola in the 1990s. Named after the town in South Africa where the accord was signed, the Kimberley Process aimed to certify diamonds at their source, with both industry representatives and participating nations agreeing not to buy or sell uncertified stones, in theory limiting armed groups' ability to use minerals for blood money. Although nations were suspended now and again for allowing illicit diamonds into their supply chains via fake certificates, and although bad actors such as Al Qaeda continue to use illicit diamonds in their transactions, the certification scheme went a long way toward creating accountability.

Yet the supply chain of jewelry diamonds is somewhat less convoluted than that of other industrial products; a mineral such as tantalum, for example, is sent to a smelter alongside minerals from other parts of the world, and refined into a single entity. When the Dodd-Frank Act passed containing Section 1502, business leaders balked at the idea that they would have to trace their products to such a minute level, for each supplier had many other suppliers, and all the streams mixed. The due diligence process for these corporations became a long backward reach, suppliers sending surveys to their suppliers, who in turn sent the same survey to their own suppliers. No one, it turned out, knew where their materials came from.

But now that the SEC was asking, they'd have to find out. The first filing was due in May of 2014. For a temporary two-year period (or four years for small businesses), companies would be allowed to classify their products as "DRC conflict undeterminable." After that, they would have to publicly assert that the products were either "DRC conflict free"—with the due diligence paperwork to prove it— or "not been found to be DRC conflict free," a designation that levied no legal charge but that opened electronics companies to the "shame and blame" strategy often used by NGOs to stir consumer backlash against those whose products are "dirty."

No single piece of foreign legislation could end the violence in the eastern Congo; beneath the issue of the mines, decades-old ethnic, political, and economic tensions simmered. But shortly after the passage of Dodd-Frank's Section 1502, Congolese president Joseph Kabila announced a ban on exports from the Walikale region, where much of the violence had unfolded. At the same time, many of the electronics industry's largest companies—having figured out which smelters tended to accept minerals from central Africa—announced they would no longer source from the eastern Congo at all. Presumably to woo those businesses back, the Congolese government announced it was backing a new minerals-tracing scheme led by the tin industry.

Six years after the passage of Dodd-Frank, it was the International Tin Association's International Tin Supply Chain Initiative (iTSCi), administered in partnership with the NGO Pact, that landed me inside that shaft on Rwanda's western edge. I'd just spent two months living outside Arusha, Tanzania, for that summer job; from there it was a cheap flight to Kigali and a three-hour hairpin-turn bus ride down to Gisenyi. In the summer of 2016, when I visited, the Cooperative COMINYABU, in Busoro, was one of 442 mines in Rwanda certified conflict free.

It was such an anonymous hill. Visible for only one bend of the road, the mine made a minor white gash in the middle of green, gray heaps of sand and mica glittering at its mouth. Beneath it, houses spread along the road like a knocked deck of cards, and the land dropped steeply into Lake Kivu.

The entrance to the shaft was fitted with a tin awning and sturdy poles of eucalyptus. Inside, wherever the mountain had shifted, jute sacks of sand pinched between scaffold and rock. The mine offered work for twelve men each day: men who descended into the dark tunnel of grit to tap at the black vein with a hammer, men who shoveled the slag upward into piles, men who broke the big rocks into dust for sale to Kigali. Each day they tagged around 150 pounds of rock.

Before sale, each bag of rock was carried up a steep slope, through tracts of banana trees and bamboo thickets, past loudly blaatting sheep, to a concrete washing station. There, with the dust flushed off and running downhill in channels, men filled sacks of rock, carefully bar-coding each one. The bar codes they used were specific to the mine and would never be used again; a poster on the wall of the Bureau de Cooperative COMINYABU down the hill reminded the miners to keep the codes locked behind two separate padlocks so they could not be stolen by smugglers.

On the one hand, the lack of conflict there was obvious. Inside the mine, men smiled shyly at me, moving aside in the dark tunnel to let me squeeze past. On their lunch breaks, they lingered beneath a copse of umusave trees, leaning easily against one another's legs. They took pictures of me with their phones when I wasn't looking, giggling if I turned in time to catch them. The men told me the money they made there was better than if they were to just cultivate the land; by mining, they could pay their children's school fees. It was, they said, "enough."

On the day I gripped the eucalyptus handrails and lowered myself into that mountain in Rwanda, following the flickers of miners' flashlights, I carried in me a vague, numb grief: I had moved so quickly from my first to my third ICD. The second defibrillator—the one that discharged a shock into itself when the wire failed and thus couldn't be trusted—inhabited my body for only the ten days between procedures, then was spirited away during the wire-removal attempt. For however intentional I'd tried to be around the global imprint of my health care, I'd been swept downstream, past my plan. The system, not me, was in charge. The hospital likely returned the ICD to St. Jude Medical as biohazard; St. Jude likely tested the electronics to see what they could learn. Then the device was likely incinerated: all that work of the planet, up in literal smoke.

As far as I'd been able to tell, there was no standardized route to managing used ICDs and pacemakers. The devices were, accidentally or intentionally, landfilled; if they outlived their owners, they sometimes exploded in the crematorium, forgotten, chipping the chimney. For this reason, some crematoriums removed them themselves, and the devices stacked up in closets as funeral home managers waited to hear back from the manufacturers about where to send them, what to do. We speak of throwing things away, but away is a place; a made object exists until destroyed. To know what it took to make a single device and then understand that it might be used only for days created a hot kind of rage in me, something wild and whiplike. I could feel viscerally the accumulation of stripped earth, of shipping containers chugging across oceans, of toxic smelters releasing their plumes, of the air-conditioning and air-filtration bills of clean rooms in Arizona and California.

The Cooperative COMINYABU, in comparison, felt good to me. Even without the ventilation and helmets and protection from cave-ins the workers would have been offered in an industrialized mine, even without health and disability insurance, this felt gentler to me somehow, like the men had access to a form of self-determination absent where warlords or corporations ruled. They were a bunch of guys with shovels and picks; their labor was their own. Other than the glittering piles at the opening of the tunnel, the mountain around us seemed intact, hardly affected. No machinery roared. Discovery of the minerals hadn't created some massive influx of diggers turning the place into a wasteland as everyone tried to get rich—as happened all over the world, at artisanal mines that sometimes caused more environmental damage than industrial operations, with no one individual or entity responsible for cleanup. And here on the Rwandan side of the border, the mineral dealers wouldn't be stopped at checkpoints to pay "taxes" to armed groups—whereas on the DRC side, the practice was rapidly gaining traction as a route to rebel financing. Even if a mine itself was conflict free, the movement of rock often lined the pockets of armed groups anyway.

Back in Kigali a few days later, the American friend I was staying with—who taught in a nursing program there—would encourage me to take whatever I'd heard with a grain of salt. She shook her head. "People will tell you what you want to hear," she said. "Things are rarely as they look in Rwanda." She meant not that I was a sucker, not that I'd been deliberately misled, but that this was how things worked, culturally. That Rwandans kept their streets clean and wore their sharpest clothes and did not criticize the government. And I saw how badly I wanted to believe that these were happy men with good lives. How badly I hoped that if we acknowledged extraction as a fundamental human activity—something every one of us did to live—we could mine in nonexploitative and life-affirming ways that left communities and forests intact.

If the story at COMINYABU were real, the coltan they dug up was the kind of metal I felt okay having in my body: metal that did not feel hot with death, heavy with suffering. Metal that did not make me wonder how my own life could possibly be worth it.

Later that night, on my friend's dripping high-rise balcony in downtown Kigali, a local artist cautioned me in the same way, as the building shook with thunder and the lights went out in the hills. "In Rwanda," he told me, "people will not tell you how they are." He was a tall, thin man with cornrowed braids that reached his shoulders, possessed of a startling depth of presence. "If they say they are great, they might not be. If they say they are just fine, then you know something is very wrong." Below us, the rain turned the roads into a silver sheen. Inside, the other party guests scooped salsa with chips and drank margaritas.

The artist and his brothers, like many Tutsi, had grown up in Uganda and come back after the genocide. They could feel the silence when they arrived, he said. How thick it was. How no one could talk about the things that had been done. The countryside in those years still smelled of the rot of bodies. The fields so full of bones the soil could not bear crops. Art was the way to see beneath those surfaces, the painter told me. Something very beautiful could be terrible inside. Something that seemed rotten might later bloom.

His work was to delicately probe the silences there. He knew the shapes and colors of them, because these were his people. They were not mine. And I wondered again how often in Madagascar I thought I had the answers I needed and abandoned the inquiry, how many times I failed to find the salient question or ask the right person or translate what I heard through a cultural lens.

In Rwanda I found a story that soothed me. The story went like this: at-the-source tagging enabled the men of Cooperative

COMINYABU to earn a good living. Through iTSCi, they were connected with corporations seeking conflict-free minerals for their products—corporations acting out the best-case scenario by actually trying, as well as they could within the framework of global capitalism, to stop funding human rights violations. For the first time we were building our ability to know, from continents away, what minerals went into a person's body.

As long as bar codes weren't slipped out of the locked cabinet. As long as bags of rocks weren't slipped in.

The story worked as long as we didn't compare the profits of corporations to what constituted a good living for the diggers.

CHAPTER 14

Tucson, Arizona
2017

For years I tried to calculate whether an implanted cardiac defibrillator was worth the cost of its creation. On one side of the ledger, I added up the village removals, the forests half cut and finally bulldozed, the lemurs crossing the road on bridges. I tallied the tailing ponds, the humming forests devoid of humans, the humans beside them desperate for work. The women kept as sex slaves in the mining slums. The women giving birth to things that were not babies.

I would never have asked the question if the device hadn't already failed me. If, as a twenty-four-year-old, I hadn't found myself septic and—after what I'd gone through to acquire an ICD—stunned by the idea that I could still die. If, at twenty-seven, I hadn't taken two thousand volts to the heart while awake, then been treated by the medical system as though this were a normal experience to have.

It was the year after the wire broke that flayed open the math for me. That rent the equation. For no matter how we treat it, a cardiac defibrillator will never stand on its own as a miracle device. The cardiac defibrillator is, and always will be, an artifact of the healthcare system administering it. It can be no more miraculous than those attending to it. It is a tool: sometimes a tool in the right hands, sometimes a tool in the wrong hands. And it is a tool particularly affected by the political winds.

* * *

By the time Donald Trump won the presidency of the United States of America late the evening of November 8, 2016, the Republican-controlled legislature had already voted to repeal the Affordable Care Act, in one form or another, eighty-three times since its passage—efforts blocked by the sitting president, Barack Obama, the man most visibly responsible for the legislation. On the morning of November 9, with a snapped wire stuck in my heart, there was room for only one thought in my head: *I will lose my health care.*

The morning after the election, as I drove north through salt flats and cotton fields toward Phoenix for a trauma sensitivity training, I called Dr. Garrick's office to make an appointment. Dr. Garrick had once suggested that his colleague in Salt Lake City, the one who'd invented the femoral procedure, might have some extra swivel in his extraction technique to dislodge the corkscrew from my heart—that maybe he could come to town to "proctor" him, in the process removing my shard in-network. Unable to access the best hospital in town because of my insurer, and unable to choose a different insurer because of the limitations of the health care marketplace, this seemed the only option worth pursuing—the only surgery that could fix the problem in my heart in-network before Donald Trump took office and inevitably signed a bill that would leave me once more uninsured. I spent my morning in class distracted, charting diagrams of how to make surgery work before the end of the year.

That evening, as I drove south back to Tucson, I took a call from my dad. "Listen," he said. "Obamacare is still the law of the land right now. If you go through open enrollment in December, you will have a contract with the insurance company for a year of coverage. Laws that get passed after January 1 will not be able to terminate your existing contract for that year. That's not how contract law works.

"And anyway, there's a lot of people who don't feel like this guy is a real Republican," he said. "We don't really know what he's going to do."

What I told myself then was: *You have one year.*

* * *

It had been six months since my wire snapped. The first time I lived with death as my constant companion, I had been twenty-four, unsure exactly what my diagnosis meant or how I was to live with it. Now I was thirty-one, and my fears were clearer. Polyurethane-silicon insulation, torn in the tugging, could flake off into the chambers of my heart. Dr. Garrick had placed the new wire out of the way of the old wire, yet I knew there was a small chance that the old one could migrate, sabotaging the new one and causing inappropriate shocks. And I feared most of all the inflammation of my tissues, the growth of scar tissue, the way my tricuspid valve could have been trashed in all the pulling. That sepsis would return and this time—with hard-to-remove hardware offering a fort for bacteria inside my heart—kill me.

Yet I was a different person from when I was twenty-four, for now I understood that death would be coming no matter what. The specifics were irrelevant. It would find all of us. Just weeks after my failed wire removal, I'd gone to Africa for my job with the global leadership organization in Tanzania. Before the start of my contract, I'd planned ten days of writing from the Kenyan coast; after, I'd tagged on my research trip to Rwanda. If in the past I justified going to the continent because I carried my own medical infrastructure, now I carried something else, too, medical detritus the nearby hospitals would not be able to do anything about. To someone like my father, this was an argument for staying home, for traveling only to places within striking distance of advanced cardiac care. But I went anyway, blearily—because I was on contract; because it was my chance to visit a mine near the DRC border; because what seemed to give my life meaning after medical failure was to stand inside a world larger than my own. The plane ticket to Nairobi my employer bought would lift me, for nearly three months, out of the buzzing Tucson heat where the wire had broken, and into a context where other questions seemed more important. This world unfolded not on fluoroscopy screens but in the smoky back alleys of Arusha, where my Tanzanian colleagues filled the table with roasted goat and cold malt soda and told stories of the brutal big game poachers. It unfolded in the long queues at clinics, sitting with whichever student worried she had an infection, harvesting "teachable moments" about the differences between health care systems. In the blur of the months after the wire broke, I introduced HIV-positive guest speakers, opened conversations on gender inequality, and discussed globalization with the groups of students who came to stay in Tengeru, a quiet village on the outskirts of Arusha. Inside the daily drama of lost cameras and packed lunches, there was little time to dwell on the changes in my body, how something essential had gone out of me in this last surgery—how before the procedure I had run nine miles up a mountain, and now two months later I lagged behind on group jogs, and struggled to hold yoga poses, and felt myself suddenly made old. I woke with my fingers pressed into the hard nub of the clot on my inner thigh. At night my co-leaders and I stayed up to sneak sips of Konyagi, a harsh Tanzanian sugarcane spirit, and talk about the other countries we'd been to, and where we would go next. I was a white American with the privilege to airlift out of her own disaster, and I had.

It was not that I was immune to worry about my own body; it was only that the worry now sat within the context of our guaranteed annihilation, the death all humans will have in a matter of time. The knowledge of it inside me felt, at turns, grainy and unreal, or desperate and electric, coming into focus at strange times—as when the Maasai elder out in the Great Rift Valley told us of their wells running dry, the walk of five miles to fill jugs. Some of us worked so hard to stay alive, and some of us didn't, or didn't yet—and every one of us would die.

How do we live in the face of the lion? We don't. If the lion is there, we must fight it or hide from it. To live with a threat constantly before us is impossible; we lash out or we coax ourselves however we can, with liquor, with social media, with oily chapati flatbread and stupid tasks. In order to live, death must take its quiet leave. To live is to forget death long enough to settle into the everyday acts of living, to believe them meaningful.

It was not a mistake to travel to East Africa that summer if I was a dying woman—and I felt like I was, though with an expiration date unknown. But it was a mistake to go if I planned to live, for the simple reason that I broke my nervous system.

To travel in East Africa that summer was to remain on high alert. On the coast south of Mombasa, where I went to write, the recent presence of the terrorist group Al-Shabaab—and reports of their interest in American nationals—altered my travel plans. A string of unrelated muggings required that I prearrange all rides. A security guard I'd flirted with tried insistently to pull me into the bushes. Even in Tengeru, where my job unfolded in a safe compound, I startled awake from roosters, loud cows, diesel generators, and rowdy students. I watched the bags, locked the windows, counted and re-counted my students in busy markets. It was a daily hypervigilance heaped onto a body that already carried the imprint of a traumatic surgery—a body already terrified of itself and what lay ahead.

At home in Arizona, I found I could not settle into quiet work. I had built for myself a brain wired for identifying and fighting threats. I blew deadlines, backed out of projects, at one point rented a hotel room an hour down the road to try to force myself into work. I had never rested after my procedures, so I never recovered. Bartending felt no easier: the crush of noise, trying to remember orders, being on my feet so long at night and so late. Scrubbing toilets in a crouch at midnight. Brushing off the comments of men. The wire seemed to glow inside me, something I remembered with a panicked jolt now and again. All that fall I rode my bike home from the bar at 1:00 a.m. with the distinct feeling that somehow my life had been lost anyway.

Though Dr. Garrick had told me there wasn't any urgency to the wire situation, I felt urgent in my body. Two months before the presidential election, when I flew to Colorado for a friend's wedding in the golden aspens, I added an appointment with Dr. Oza to my schedule. Even though he'd played a critical role in convincing me to receive an ICD I now had deep doubts about, I never blamed him. He seemed to make decisions carefully, and I knew he truly cared about me and my sister. He'd donated his surgical fee and advocated on my behalf. For my own mental health I needed to sit face-to-face with an electrophysiologist who would look me in the eye.

I'd last seen Dr. Oza at the farmer's market four years earlier, the spring I made the decision to leave town for graduate school; we'd found ourselves next to each other in the bread line. Then, his face had noticeably fallen when I told him I was leaving Boulder. Now, he opened the door to the exam room with a smile.

After the pleasantries, he asked, "Why have you come to see me?" He'd received my records. "I am not an expert on wire removal."

"I know," I told him. I shared my nagging feeling that Dr. Garrick was suggesting the Salt Lake City expert come down to Tucson so that Dr. Garrick could learn from my rare case rather than because it was my best medical option. I asked Dr. Oza whom he would send me to if it were his decision, and he recommended a lead extraction special-ist at the Cleveland Clinic. Dr. Oza also confirmed that my fears of insulation flaking off the wire were not entirely unfounded; there weren't many patients in my exact situation to compare me to.

At the end, he regarded me seriously. "I'm sorry this happened to you," he said, and my eyes filled with tears.

"Thank you," I said.

It was this, as much as anything else, that I had come for.

By the spring of 2017, as Donald Trump assumed the presidency, the most powerful person in my world was a woman named Jenny. As Dr. Garrick's assistant, Jenny was the one tasked with keeping the ball rolling on this surgeon's visit to Tucson. Though I'd wanted to follow Dr. Oza's advice and connect with the lead extraction specialist at the Cleveland Clinic, the cardiologist he'd recommended wasn't covered by my insurance network. A surgery there would either be prohibi-tively expensive or logistically messy. The plan involving Dr. Garrick's colleague from Salt Lake seemed the fastest and least expensive route to removing my wire before the political winds whisked my health care away.

It was hard to know how often to follow up with Jenny that spring; was she truly working on it, or had she forgotten? Back in November, she advised me to get on Dr. Garrick's schedule to speed the process along, even though I required no medical advice from him at the time; a $50 copay later, I'd leave without any new knowledge, just the hope that they would keep managing my case when I was not in front of them. I called and called. "Jenny, it's Kati Standefer," I'd say into her voice-mail in-box. "I'm trying to figure out when I can teach. Do you know the surgery dates yet?" This, again and again, my calls becoming more insistent, my panic rising as the Republican-held legislature debated more seriously plans to repeal the Affordable Care Act.

Finally, there was a date range; the surgeon would be in for a conference in early May. Jenny booked me an appointment with Dr. Garrick during which the surgeon would be present to consult. If it seemed like a fit, we could then book the surgery center for a few days later. It was a relief to have something, anything, on the calendar.

"Hey! I've got a question for you!"

By the time the man in the black pickup pulled over to shout at us, the protest was almost over, a raggedy line of people in the ninety-degree March sun, mostly elderly and white, donning sun hats and visually categorizable as "granola." In early January of 2017— before Donald Trump had taken office and just days after the House of Representatives began voting to repeal the Affordable Care Act— a man in an SUV had turned left into my car, totaling it. I'd struggled to find a new car I could afford in the midst of a busy winter, and the man's skimpy insurance policy and unresponsiveness left me without a rental. On this day, then, I'd ridden my bike the seven miles uphill into the foothills in north Tucson on a Friday afternoon to join the protest at Senator Jeff Flake's office. I knew I wouldn't forgive myself if I lost my health care without doing everything in my power to prevent it.

The gathering felt more symbolic than functional. Senator Flake's office complex was technically private property, so we were relegated to protesting at its entrance, on the dusty side of a busy road, out of sight of his staff. From time to time people stashed their signs and traipsed in to register public comments, an excuse to enter his air-conditioned waiting room.

"If that building was built after 1990, I'm gonna sue his ass," a white-haired woman in a sun hat beside me had remarked when I came down from registering my official opposition to the American Health Care Act, the House Republicans' first serious attempt at repealing and replacing the Affordable Care Act. The woman wore a green plaid shirt and sat in an electric wheelchair, with a SAVE OUR HEALTH CARE sign propped in her lap. She told me there hadn't been an accessibility button on the door, as required by the Americans with Disabilities Act. She had to bang on the glass doors until someone heard her and let her in.

"Zika virus," she told me without my asking, smoothing her white pants. Ten years earlier she'd lost use of both legs. She told me she lived in the West University neighborhood downtown. "I've figured out I have enough juice to get me to Representative Grijalva's office," she said, "and then I recharge my chair at the library before heading home."

I'd seen the man in the big black truck pulling over before I heard his voice, and instinctively started walking toward him. I found myself deeply moved by some of the protesters, such as this woman with Zika, picturing her making the long buzzing trek downtown in her wheelchair. Others I found myself weary of. They did not seem particularly representative of the intersectional movement I claimed as my own, and many of the posters they held that day seemed vaguely hysterical, imprecise, the messages unlikely to change the mind of anyone who wasn't already going to beep his horn for us.

The posters could, in fact, make someone mad enough to pull over, and now I found myself walking faster to edge out a thin man with a white mustache who was also approaching the black truck. I'd worked hard to learn about health-care policy. It felt like my turn.

"I've got a question for you," the man said again, hollering from the driver's seat with his passenger window open. "I've worked since I was fourteen. Never stopped since."

"What makes you think we haven't been working since we were fourteen, too?" I couldn't help saying, laughing, and he cut me off.

"Just listen," he said. He told us how since the passage of the Affordable Care Act, his premium had tripled. He told us that last year in order to pay his taxes he had to pull money out of his IRA, and as a result his subsidy went down. Then he furiously pulled down the edge of his shirt, a short, thin scar running over his pectoral.

"And I have a pacemaker!" he proclaimed.

I pulled down the edge of my tank top to show him the pale pink scar below my own collarbone. "Me, too!" I said.

At this, he stopped. His face changed. "Really," he said. "Look at that."

"A defibrillator, actually," I said.

"Aren't you young?" he said, his voice no longer loud.

"We have a genetic arrhythmia in my family," I told him. He shook his head.

"I even have a broken wire stuck in my heart," he said, his face betraying worry now.

"Me, too!" I hooted, and at this we both laughed, incredulous. "Sir, we are the same," I said. "I just happen to make less money—I'm a writer—so I get a better subsidy. I wouldn't be able to access health care without the Obamacare marketplace and these subsidies. I'm lucky. But you're right in the worst spot in the subsidy structure of the ACA. Obamacare is not perfect, and it could use some fixes."

He was listening now.

"But what the Republicans have proposed won't fix that problem," I said. He was watching me carefully. "I would support a bill that fixed the problems of Obamacare, but this isn't it," I said, our eyes locked.

"I guess I just felt like you were protesting *me*," the man said, and for the second time I could see his worry, the anger atop it draining off.

"We're not protesting you," I said. "We've been lucky to be helped by Obamacare. We're protesting a bill that doesn't fix its problems. We're on your side."

He shrugged, gave a half wave, and drove off.

What Jenny giveth, Jenny taketh away.

The surgeon had learned there would be a fee for him to practice out of state in a network and facility not his own. I'd always assumed there would be such a fee and that he found my case fascinating enough to brush off the cost, or that perhaps Dr. Garrick would absorb it as part of his "proctoring." Instead, Jenny told me the surgeon would attend the conference but not see me in Arizona. "The whole team" would have to travel to Salt Lake.

To travel to Salt Lake City to see this surgeon would require an out-of-network authorization, and if I had that, there was no need for Dr. Garrick's involvement beyond the paperwork. In the furious, panicked days that followed Jenny's call, as I pedaled and pedaled around town, as I cleared glasses from tables during my job at the beer bar, an idea filtered into my mind, then solidified. If I needed an out-of-network authorization anywhere—with the increased risk of something not being covered and roaring in at full cost out-of-pocket—I would use it to get to the best: Dr. Michael Ackerman of the Mayo Clinic, a pediatric cardiologist known to be one of the world's foremost experts on long QT.

I would not just ask a top-level cardiologist to remove my wire. I would finally steer into the nagging question at the back of my mind: whether I had ever needed an ICD in the first place.

I'd met Dr. Ackerman in November, the week before the election, at Tucson's Fox Theatre for a talk he was giving as part of the Andra Heart Speaker Series—organized by the parents of a twelve-year-old girl named Andra Dalrymple who'd died suddenly from undiagnosed long QT in 2010. When the event invite landed in my in-box at the University of Arizona College of Medicine, where I was teaching in a narrative medicine pilot for first-year medical students, I'd stared at it in delight. Dr. Ackerman was someone I'd heard about for years. He was the president of SADS, the advocacy organization I'd reached out to when I was trying to determine how dangerous exercise was, and he directed the Mayo Clinic's Long QT Syndrome/Genetic Heart Rhythm Clinic and the Windland Smith Rice Sudden Death Genomics Laboratory in Rochester, Minnesota. Now here he was in Tucson—giving both an evening public talk on sudden cardiac death prediction and prevention in the young and, the next day, a more technical talk about genetics at the medical school.

He would also be meeting with faculty by appointment.

I arrived alone and too early to Dr. Ackerman's talk at the Fox, filling my plate with free tamales, standing by myself at a tall table in the foyer to eat. Two women edged toward my table. "Do you mind if we join you?" one of them said. Then she looked at me again. "Oh," she said, "you have an essay in *Best American Essays 2016,* right?"

"I do," I said, flushing, pleased and surprised.

"My husband and I saw your reading the other night," she said. "It was great."

"That's so lovely," I said. "Thanks for coming."

The woman introduced herself as Bridget. Her husband, she told me, was also a pediatric cardiologist, a professor of pediatrics at the university. He would be escorting Dr. Ackerman. Not long after, her husband, Brent, arrived at the table, tall, boyish, and brown-haired, with a balding Dr. Ackerman in tow. Brent did a double take when he saw me.

"Hey!" he said, delight evident on his face. "We saw you read the other night, didn't we?" He turned to Dr. Ackerman. "This is—"

"Kati Standefer," I said, holding out my hand.

"She has an essay in *Best American Essays 2016*, and we heard her read on Friday," Brent said.

"Well, fabulous," Dr. Ackerman said, beaming his wide, slightly gapped grin at me. There was a sweetness in him visible immediately. "What's the essay about?"

"Yeah, what's the essay about, Kati?" Bridget said, holding back a smile. A blush crept up Brent's neck.

"Well," I said, "It's about me having sex with a married man I don't particularly like, a sort of manifesto about our right to sexual pleasure even if we are single long-term."

Dr. Ackerman laughed in a slightly awkward, decidedly midwestern sort of way. "Maybe you should take the stage instead," he said. "That sounds much more interesting than what I'm about to say."

"I'm sure that's not true," I said. "We're actually meeting tomorrow. I teach narrative medicine at the college of medicine. But I'm here tonight as a long QT patient. Type 2."

At this his face shifted. He tipped his head. "And I don't know you yet?" In the tender edge to his voice I understood he had a large, widespread flock tucked beneath his wings. There weren't many of us—researchers estimate that around one in 2,500 people are affected by a genetic long QT—and even fewer emerge symptomatic. But when one of us does emerge, the effect ripples through families, and many of them land in Dr. Ackerman's clinic.

When it was time to settle into the auditorium, I wandered into one of the front rows. Dr. Ackerman, fiddling with his mike, called down to me. "Are you sure you don't want to come up here instead?" he said. "The stage is ready for you!" I laughed, shook my head.

Dr. Ackerman had a dorky playfulness to him; his earnest midwesternness seemed, up until that point, to be his overriding feature. But as the lights went down and his slide show went up, I could suddenly feel the force of his intelligence. As he spoke it became clear that he was not simply an activist physician; he was systematically using his research team to fill gap after gap in what the world knew about sudden arrhythmia death syndromes, including long QT. With each study result came a more refined next question, and as the results accrued, so did our ability to predict how the different types of long QT would act and to thus filter out, for each type, the treatment methods that weren't as effective. The man had published more than four hundred articles. I could see that while any number of electrophysiologists might be good at their jobs in the abstract, he was one of the few driving the conversation around long QT, which meant it was other electrophysiologists' job to keep up with his research. And did they? We young adults with long QT formed a tiny percentage of cardiac patients compared to the masses of elderly heart-failure patients who poured into cardiologists' offices. What was the likelihood that a given doctor had seen the latest findings from Dr. Ackerman and his team? What did it mean to be a good long QT doctor?

At that moment, out of a weird intuition, I turned around to scan the audience. I saw, a few rows behind me, the face of Dr. Garrick.

It was as if I had run into someone who was at once a lover and a rapist. Someone who I had trusted, who had been inside my body, who had tugged at the most intimate, central part of me. Someone under whose watch a horrible thing had unfolded.

A jolt ran through my body. A compulsion and a repulsion. I had seen him only once since the wire broke, and I wanted to stare. I wanted to hide.

He was at least in the room with the research, I told myself. But I knew that was only part of being a good doctor.

* * *

The next morning, I met Dr. Ackerman in a glass-walled room in the Sarver Heart Center at Banner–University Medical Center. I told him that, as someone who worked in the field of narrative medicine, I was curious how he built the story of long QT for his patients—especially because so many of them were children, their lives so shaped by their early illness.

"The philosophy is, *Thou shalt live and thrive,*" said Dr. Ackerman, crossing his long legs and leaning back. "That sets the tone, sets the atmosphere. One of my first questions for my patients is, What do you love?

"This is a very different approach from the mainstream," he said. "My role isn't to kick people out of anything. The fundamental role of the physician is to be the Great Adviser, not the Gestapo." Young people are paying attention, Dr. Ackerman said. They pick up on a physician's confidence. And they think, *If all these things have to be censored from my life, death is around the corner.* That sense isn't always irrational; young long QT patients have sometimes just lost siblings. They've gone into cardiac arrest in gymnasiums and been resuscitated by coaches doing chest compressions. But what research tells us is that long QT is unlikely to kill those who know they have it; being able to manage the condition generally prevents sudden cardiac death. What Dr. Ackerman tells kids is: "Badness is not going to strike you.

"A lot of times, the kids don't say a lot," he said. "They're listening, trusting. Mom, Dad, and the doctor know what they're doing. There's a quietness there. They're defaulting to others' expertise. Then on the flight home, they ask, 'What's my risk?'

"We start with, 'We probably won't need a device,'" Dr. Ackerman said. "You don't need a sledgehammer for a tack nail." His clinic at Mayo only includes an ICD in treatment plans around 20 percent of the time, and this rate includes devices other practitioners have placed. Though Dr. Ackerman has long consulted for the major device manufacturers—Boston Scientific, Medtronic, St. Jude Medical—he told me he continues to ask himself, "Why do I feel like I must implant? I'm a genetic cardiologist, not an ICD specialist. I'm not wedded to any particular treatment. I'm wedded to the patient."

He once counted that he had patients on around twenty different permutations of treatment plans.

"We would be using devices a whole lot more if they lasted forever and nothing went wrong with them," he continued. "People have not appreciated the baggage that comes with defibrillator care." Frayed leads, battery recalls, the size of the device, unnecessary shocks.

"What is your sense of the S-ICD as a response to some of these problems?" I asked him.

"I don't love it yet," he said. While the lack of wires in the heart makes it potentially less damaging, he said, he felt the incorrect shock rate was still too high in long QT patients.

That morning was the first time I had heard a doctor use the term "beta-blocker zombie." It was the first time I heard a doctor acknowledge that when patients feel disconnected they become high-maintenance, and that what doctors say—or don't say—can create a sense of death lurking. It was the first time I heard a doctor acknowledge that when patients feel their doctors are truly on their team, the way they manage their mortality changes.

"If you are not happy with the quality of your life, we've got a problem," Dr. Ackerman said.

When it came time for us to go into the other room and fill our plates with Mediterranean food, Dr. Ackerman cueing his genomics slide show for the cardiology department, I wanted to cover my face in my hands and weep.

I found my doctor.

In an ideal health-care system, one might call and make an appointment. One might then go.

In the health-care system in which I found myself, calling the Long QT Syndrome/Genetic Heart Rhythm Clinic at Mayo to schedule appointments proved only the beginning. For an out-of-network authorization is a version of hell in which one's effort can be entirely disconnected from outcome.

There is no moment at which anyone explains the process to you. It took a while before I understood where to begin and what I must do. Although Dr. Garrick agreed it was a good idea that I both see a specialist about removing the wire and consult with Dr. Ackerman about managing my long QT going forward, in practical terms getting his office to actually complete and submit the authorization request to my insurance company proved nightmarish. Mayo booked a number of tests automatically as part of my consultation, and each of these had to be specifically mentioned on the preapproval paperwork or I could be liable for its cost, and—since I would never see this paperwork myself—ideally this meant that Mayo and Pima Heart would communicate with each other.

Too late I realized this would not happen. I stepped out of a bar shift one afternoon to accept a call from Rochester, Minnesota, and learned that it was the Mayo Clinic billing office calling because they didn't have prior authorization yet from my insurance company—which they would need before my arrival, or they would turn me into a "self-pay" patient and require a $5,000 deposit before I could receive services. The appointment dates roared toward us. Already my flight had been booked, the hotel and the shuttle from Minneapolis to Rochester; my parents would meet me in Minnesota by car, and if I had surgery to remove the wire they would bring me home to Illinois with them to rest. Now I raced the clock, making the calls over and over—to my insurance company to see if the paperwork had gone in, to Jenny to find out the billing codes they were using, to Mayo's billing office to make sure they had all the codes. Insert here the hours on hold with my insurance company, the attempt to figure out if any tests would likely *not* be approved out of network so I could have them in-network right before I flew to Mayo. Insert here the business hours slipping by, my freelance work ignored, my ability to earn a living diminishing with every day as I managed my health care full-time. In these same weeks I was trying to buy a car, increasingly frantic as car after car fell through, worried that, if my heart tore during the removal, I would arrive home with a freshly stitched sternum and find only my bike as transportation. Meanwhile the House of Representatives blustered about and tweaked and finally passed the American Health Care Act, a bill that did not explicitly end my access to health care but that repealed the taxes that paid for the Affordable Care Act's subsidies, slashed cost-sharing payments that made insurance affordable for people like me, ended the Medicaid expansion program that had given me insurance out of graduate school, did away with the individual and employer mandates that stabilized the market, ended Obama-era rules capping how much insurance companies could charge people with preexisting conditions, and allowed states to waive basic essential coverage standards, all of which the Congressional Budget Office predicted would cause twenty-four million people—including, probably, me—to lose health insurance by 2026, potentially starting the so-called death spiral Republican politicians loved to refer to that spring, in which insurers would simply choose not to offer their services on the original ACA marketplaces and Obamacare could be called dead.

Somewhere in these weeks, I began to scream at people on the phone.

"If you've had open heart surgery, you will wake with your hands tied and a breathing tube in," my friend Janelle said gently, her spoon scraping a cup of chocolate peanut butter ice cream. It had been almost a year since my wire broke. On this hot afternoon in early May a few weeks before I was supposed to leave for Mayo, she'd picked me up and driven us to the north end of town, where in a nondescript strip mall there was a new ice cream shop we wanted to try. We sat outside the front door of the shop, facing the parking lot and the mountains. "It's good to know that going in. It's likely you will have an IV in your neck. When you get the tube out, you will gag."

Tall, with wavy brown hair and a generous laugh, Janelle had lived in the casita behind my house for two years before moving in with her now-husband. She was a nurse in University Medical Center's cardiac ICU. Knowing that my wire removal had already failed once, I understood that the risk of the heart tissue tearing was real, and I'd asked her to help me prepare for what could be coming.

"If you wake up intubated," she said, taking a bite, "you'll feel like you can't get enough air. You can practice the feeling by breathing through a straw. Actually, you do yoga—so practice open-chest poses before going in. You can roll up a yoga mat and place it under your shoulder blades, to stretch out before surgery. It will be the last time you can do that for a while, and you'll want to go in strong."

When we booked the ice cream date, I told her I felt like I didn't know what questions to ask my doctors. Now she rattled them off. "Are you at increased risk for clotting from what is attaching to the wire, that could break off and cause a stroke? Are you going to be intubated and sedated either way? How will you wake up, and what will you wake up to? Will you go to a cardiac ICU or a normal ICU? Will your ICD be turned on or off? How soon can your parents be with you? Where can they be with you, and where can't they come? Who will be in communication with them?" She told me to bring a small dry-erase board with markers, and a notebook and pen, so we could keep track of the comings and goings, so I could ask questions while intubated.

Bleeds, she told me, come in different forms. The risk wasn't just a flood of blood that could keep the heart from pumping. Slow bleeds were a problem, too. They'd monitor for that, she said; they could put in a chest tube to prevent tamponade.

"The chest tubes rub around in there," she said. "They'll put lidocaine patches by the chest tube insertion site. They'll stay there for the bleeding two to three days, tops. They'll do an aseptic chest preparation, but yes, it can be an infection site. You'll wear masks—you, the nurse, everyone. You will be *exhausted*. But we lose aerobic fitness in just seventy-two hours, and the first morning without your tube you *must* go to the chair. Patients do as well as they are willing to do. They have to put in the effort of breathing, coughing, walking. You're the ideal patient, though. You're an otherwise healthy adult. You have intact skin and strong muscles."

"Intact skin?" I wrinkled my nose. "Jesus."

"Yeah," she widened her eyes, "those are the patients in real trouble.

"Surgery is an intentional injury to the body," she said, crossing her long legs. "It might help to think of it that way. You will have essentially been through a bad car crash, only for a better reason."

Ask why things are being done. Ask the purpose of medications. Ask them to make sure the sheath is out this time before you're awake. If an alarm goes off, ask what it's for and what they're going to do about it, and if they're not going to do anything, get the parameters changed so it's not jangling all night long.

Tell the staff: even if Kati looks asleep, she wants to be told what you're going to do before anything happens.

Tell your parents to hold your hand even if it's tied.

By then I was brittle with despair. It had been a year that proved to me how little of our lives we actually control, that one could spend years at a time asserting her will without anything coming of it. One could receive medical treatment that was supposed to save her life but instead endangered it. One could be hit by a car on a normal Saturday evening, on the way home from a trailhead; one could begin a promising relationship and then never hear from him again; one could dial Congress every day and see the news becoming ever worse; one could waste entire days on the phone with insurance companies and hospitals without things ever being arranged; one could attempt to buy car after car and still end the day on a bike. One could spend so much time on all this that her career falls apart.

The risk of the procedure—of death—loomed before me. Unlike the previous year, when the threat of death sharpened my resolve to do the things I loved, now the dull march toward death in a surgical theater rendered everything pointless. I was spending all my time fighting for something that carried a statistically significant risk of ending me—and so meaninglessness stretched out forward and behind.

To live seemed suddenly a stupid sort of faith, a treadmill of activity without meaning or reward.

It was as if a veil had suddenly pulled back before me: if the reasons we have for living are the things and people we love most, all of these too can be lost. A brutal end awaits our bodies, which we will lose in stages, and a brutal end awaits everyone we love, possible every moment. To say this has become a cliché, but to know it viscerally is something else altogether, a horror perhaps beyond any other. One cannot come to this place and not be changed by it. If all our efforts are for those who will become corpses, if the books we write will somewhere rot, the whole project of living is absurd.

Once one arrives in this place, one can either choose to live, or not. We have to tell ourselves a story that makes living possible. God is one such story, that we live because a creator wants us to, because there is some master plan for us. Or we live for our children, whose lives somehow supersede ours in significance. I had neither kids nor god, and wanted neither. I had no partner carrying a shared vision. I found myself dangerously unmoored, swaying in the hot winds of whatever phone calls unfolded that day, disconnected from anything that mattered except for my friends, showing up in their quiet ways, dropping me at medical appointments on the other side of town or lending me their cars or arriving at the beer bar with dinner to share on my break, listening, always, to the ranting, formless stories that had come to comprise my life.

"Living, naturally, is never easy," writes Albert Camus in *The Myth of Sisyphus*. "You continue making the gestures commanded by existence for many reasons, the first of which is habit. Dying voluntarily implies that you have recognized, even instinctively, the ridiculous character of that habit, the absence of any profound reason for living, the insane character of that daily agitation and the uselessness of suffering."

But what had begun did not stop. Jenny, I finally learned in one of my calls, had submitted the prior authorization to the wrong insurance company, my insurer from the *previous* year. I wasn't sure how it had happened. I only knew that the window had almost closed on finalizing my prior authorization at Mayo. I called. I called. I called.

Jenny resubmitted late, without ten business days left until the appointment.

There was one last chance, the insurance company told me, after a message, after a long hold. The referring doctor could check an Urgent box to expedite the prior-authorization form. It was at Dr. Garrick's discretion; if he checked it, they would rush it. Period. I put the call in to Jenny.

He declined.

I would not lose life or limb, Jenny told me, and that's what "urgent" meant to him. It was a medical judgment.

But once more our version of medicine proved blind to what I was losing.

If this story of a woman's preauthorization feels laborious and a bit annoying, that's because it is. The bureaucracy of a preauthorization is profoundly boring, except, of course, when it is connected to your very life—when you think, as I did, that this may be the last year in which you will have access to insurance, when you think it is your last chance to remove from your body an object of medical detritus you know will prove a problem on some distant day, and when you already know, as I did, exactly what it feels like to have no health insurance on the day something goes wrong.

If the story of a preauthorization seems like a lot of meaningless back-and-forth, it is: only it is a meaninglessness that becomes one's life. In such a battle with health-care bureaucracy, the hours of mean-inglessness grow tumorously, crowding out other uses of one's talents and time, wrecking some of the reasons to live even as it is living one fights for. One becomes hypervigilant, waiting to dial the moment business hours open, tracking the last time one called lest one later be blamed. One can throw at a problem all the hours she has and see no reward for her attempts; one can even be, as I was, college-educated and deeply experienced in the insurance system and still feel like Sisyphus, rolling a rock up a hill only to watch it roll back down.

The system is not built to deliver care. It is built to maximize profit, not only by denying care but by frustrating patients until they quit trying. The system is built not for patients but for the profit engines of pharmaceutical companies, medical device manufacturers, and "not-for-profit" hospitals that set high prices to pay their executives millions. In the middle sit insurance companies, trying to pay as little of these extraordinary costs as possible—protecting themselves from paying out their profits. They protect themselves not only at the price of our health, but at the price of our sanity.

Not only had the defibrillator not saved my life with its shocks; not only had it gone from being a technology of promise to a flapping de-tritus bearing new complications; not only had it been forged at such ecological and social cost; now the process of trying to get appropriate care for what was stranded inside me had so ruined my quality of life that I wanted to be dead. If the *causa finalis* of a defibrillator is the need to prevent premature death in a young woman with a genetic condition, the ICD—within this system—is broken.

"In life as in story," writes Arthur Frank, "one event is expected to lead to another." Our medical system has sold us a story of remedy, progress, technology, professionalism, and triumph. Frank suggests that our society is willing to hear only those illness narratives that conform to the idea of "restitution": *I was well, I got sick, I am well again.* "It's nothing," we insist before a procedure, knowing that medicine will shortly deliver a triumph. "I'm fine," we say afterward, as though nothing has fundamentally shifted inside us. We crave the clean plot arc, one those around us can understand and stomach. When we try to tell the story of the phone calls, pointless and insane, our listeners lean away.

And yet we cannot separate individual treatments, however sophisticated, from the system in which they are rendered, if that system is providing not safety and care but frustration, futility, and impotence. If that system creates experiences that look less like restitution and more like what Frank calls chaos narratives.

"In the chaos narrative, troubles go all the way down to bottomless depths," writes Frank. "What can be told only begins to suggest all that is wrong. The second feature of the chaos narrative...is the syntactic structure of 'and then and then and then.'...

"The lack of any coherent sequence is an initial reason why chaos stories are hard to hear;...they are threatening. The anxiety these stories provoke inhibits hearing....The story traces the edges of a wound that can only be told around....In the lived chaos there is no mediation, only immediacy. The body is imprisoned in the frustrated needs of the moment."

Chaos narratives, writes Frank, expose the fundamental contingency at the heart of living, all the ways we cannot control our bodies or our lives, all the ways our lives can be wasted, and they are, for this reason, unbearable.

Then we were approaching summer. With kids off school it was harder for the Long QT Syndrome Clinic to fit me in. The scheduler called, finally, with new appointments spread out over four days in early June, with a weekend in between Day 1 and Day 2. I said yes; I had to. I'd finally bought a truck, a little red 2004 Nissan Frontier. I would drive, I decided, for dexterity. The calendar was blank. I would put my body in the Midwest and be ready.

The night before I began my drive to the Mayo Clinic, I got off at the bar at 10:00 p.m. and drove the wide, empty streets to Sabino Canyon. In a few weeks, when the heat really settled into Tucson, this parking lot would be busy at all hours, marathon runners arriving at 3:00 and 4:00 a.m. to train under the cover of darkness. But, on this night, the place was empty at 10:15 p.m.—just me under the scrap of the moon, a few bats wheeling beneath the parking-lot lights. I slipped on my running shoes and belt of water, and set out down the dark trail with the single beam of my phone light bouncing before me.

By the time this moon was full I would be two thousand miles from here; after all these months working out the logistics, whether or not the appointments were fully authorized, I would finally drive away toward heart surgery. I did not know how many runs I had left in my life. I did not know when and in what condition I would return to my desert home.

It was hard to keep pace in the dark: the uncertain footfalls, a spray of pebbles now and then, the awareness of cacti at the edge and the snakes who might drape their bodies across the trail. It wasn't long before I turned off my phone light, took out my earbuds, and slowed to a walk.

It takes time for the eyes to adjust to darkness, I thought, reaching the place where the trail crossed the road. It takes time to adjust to the rough shape of things. But I found the trail. Walking with little light was what I had been practicing all those months.

The saguaros stood sentinel with their dark spring hats of flowers. My body could discern the landing of a bird from the rustle of javelinas, but it had not evolved to manage the graveyard of metal and plastic that now sat in the center of me, this thing that was simultaneously threat and not threat. It had been a long time since I walked like this, and of course it was unsensible: to end a bar shift with a night hike in a place where spiky things reigned, on a simmering hundred-degree night. The next day, I had a long drive ahead of me.

Still, it struck me that part of what I lost in that season of insurance phone calls, those five months without a car, had been this sustenance, a connection with what was older and wiser than I. I thought of the mine sites on the other side of the world, the communities told they could not return to the places of their ancestors or the homes they had known. I found myself remembering, all at once, a night in my cabin in Hoback when I'd walked out the door into a lightless blizzard, comforted by the press of snow against my thighs. How I'd walked toward the river, heard a heavily laden pine branch drop snow with a *whoosh*.

I used to always know the stages of the moon if you asked me, and that night when I finally turned back, the curve of it hanging there, high and bright, confronted me like an old lover, who holds the truths of a past life.

Faintly now: the smell of water.

I did not need to look down then. I trusted my feet, trusted the instincts of my body. I put my arms out, aware that stumbling is a part of being alive, glad for the earth beneath me. The light, for the first time in a long time, seemed enough.

CAUSA EFFICIENS

CHAPTER 15

Rochester, Minnesota
2017

The Mayo Clinic was a cathedral of kindness, designed for light and quiet. The eastern flank of the Gonda Building, where cardiology was housed, rose in a wall of windows. Inside the building's entrance, a three-story curving canyon opened, gleaming wood lining each level, an atrium where people clustered quietly to hear a small girl play gorgeous, precise violin.

I had expected a sprawling white campus, with the same low ceilings and rows of waiting-room chairs and endless parking lots I had seen in medical offices across the country. I had expected an air of misery about the place, all those bald scalps and wheelchairs, the sickest patients in the world disembarking after a string of medical failures, but instead when we arrived late at night I'd noticed the quiet beauty of the Kahler Grand Hotel, the particular kindness of the clerks. This would turn out to be true everywhere in town. At the desk where I checked in for my exercise treadmill test, I saw a small scrap of paper taped to the counter, facing the receptionist: "Be kind, for everyone you meet is fighting a great battle."

To work at Mayo must put one so close to the edge, I thought, must require one to stare into the void on the regular.

Elsewhere, this meant a hardening. Here, it meant cultivating softness.

* * *

I'd spent the afternoon of my thirty-second birthday fighting with my insurance company and the Mayo billing office, driving through the green hills of Iowa at eighty miles per hour. For three days there had been a reprieve. I'd driven up the belly of Arizona, headed east across New Mexico, camped on the side of a mountain in Colorado. I'd barreled through Kansas to eat barbecue with an old friend just over the Missouri border, and, in the morning, cut north. Though initially I'd been told that the now-preauthorized appointments operated as an umbrella—meaning any code the physician might order relating to the visit would be covered—just west of Iowa City I received a call from the Mayo billing office telling me one of the largest codes did not fall under that umbrella and had been left off the form. I would need to provide $5,000 up front in order to be seen in a few days.

When I hung up I screamed and screamed into the cab of the truck. My hand itched to crank the wheel. I pictured green rushing up to meet me before the shatter of glass. The blank of concrete accordioning the vehicle. My insides all metal.

By the end of the day, I would have a supervisor from Mayo's billing office working on the issue with Dr. Garrick's office, going through code by code to make sure they were all submitted. It was the accountability I had been looking for all this time. Now, since the final codes were submitted but not authorized, the question was whether we would have to cancel Friday's appointments. If I went before they were authorized and the permission was granted afterward, everything would be retroactively covered—it might be worth going anyway—but Mayo's policy of requiring $5,000 up front for anything unauthorized hung over my head. It was money I didn't have. If I canceled, it could be weeks before the Long QT Clinic could fit me in again.

When I finally arrived in Illinois at dusk, puffy-eyed and weary, everyone was waiting in the kitchen; my parents, my older sister, Cindy, who lived in town, even Christine, who lived in Denver. My father poured me a whiskey. Candles crowded my birthday cake: a 9, an 8, a 7, a 5, and three slender singles pushed into the chocolate frosting. The math was right—thirty-two—but it looked like 9,875, and I nearly cried laughing looking at it, how old I felt.

The consultations I'd worked for were finally so close. Yet some crucial tautness had loosened in me; ends flapped. I no longer knew what to do with a life. And so three days later, on a Thursday afternoon, my college best friend, Makendra, flew into O'Hare, her thick curly dark hair stashed beneath a cap. Eight years earlier, she had co-signed on my Boulder apartment via shoddy Wyoming fax machine. Seven years earlier, she had arrived into my first sepsis hospital room as my mom headed home, and smoothed warm blankets over me after I threw up. Now, she would drive northwest to Mayo with me, since my parents had a wedding to attend in Illinois over the weekend. While I had tests done, Mak would wait, twisting wire into the bitty horses she sold at small shops. Then we would drive to Red Wing—a tiny town pressed up against the Mississippi River that once birthed an eponymous line of boots—to spend the weekend between my appointments. We would hike the steep bluff that towered over town. We would read in bed, drink pints in the old brewing district, watch barges push down the river at dusk. But Mak's main job was to keep me from walking off a latticed bridge into the swirling brown waters. To keep me in the world of the living.

We loaded the car. Not knowing whether I would have surgery before I returned, I said goodbye to the house I grew up in. I said goodbye to the dog. Christine followed me out to the car. "What are you thinking?" she said.

"I want to die," I said, aware that it made no sense, that the whole Mayo trip was an act against death. Still, death had cohabited my body too long; it twisted in me and surrounded me. The taste of cardboard in my mouth. "I feel like I should be going with you," Christine said mournfully. "It feels weird that you're going first."

At the Illinois-Wisconsin border I saw that Mayo had called. When I got Brad, the billing manager, back on the line, he told me they tried to get Dr. Garrick to check the Urgent box on the billing code that had been left off. Again he'd refused, insisting it wasn't medically urgent. Panic gripped my throat, the taillights around us beginning to blur.

"We are on our *way*," I began, and Makendra looked over in alarm. "We are on 90 right now—"

"I know," Brad said. I squeezed the wheel. Bugs clotted the windshield, sticking to the wipers like hardened jam. "Listen, this one time, we won't ask you to pay up front. We have confirmation that it's in the pipeline and I know you've done all you can. The cost will be yours if it doesn't authorize," he said, "but having talked to everyone involved, we don't see a reason it wouldn't."

I cried into the heel of my hand, trying to keep the car in its narrow lane, stunned by this simple kindness. Beside me, Makendra quietly pulled out her homemade cookies, and set one on my knee. We drove north, then west, tailing the sunset, the green Midwest clicking and humming around us. The moon rising over the empty truck bed.

And then, after all that time and work, there I was, sitting in Dr. Ackerman's exam room. For what it had taken to get there, the room felt strangely normal, unextraordinary: an examination table, a desk with a computer, the floor a pebbly-looking brown laminate. Out the window, the afternoon was dark. Rain shuddered sideways against the glass. I'd finished my testing: a second ECG by a woman who remembered me from the first; the electrodes of a Holter monitor stickered onto my chest and its plastic recorder tucked into my breasts for twenty-four hours of observation; an appointment with cardiology's genetic counselor, which began with a nurse introducing me to the front-desk staff, each of them leaning across the counter to shake my hand, smiling at me. "They will all help you," the nurse said, "and they will visit you when you are in the hospital."

At the genetics consultation, the counselor had stopped in the doorway. "Dr. Ackerman likes to say hi if he's here, even though your appointment is later," she said. "Is that okay?"

"Of course," I said, and she ducked her head back out, and within minutes his tall frame came through the door.

He reached out his hand, smiling, and then at once tilted his head. "I know you," he said.

"We met in Tucson," I said, and his face lit with recognition.

"Yes!" A pause. "The essay." Both of us cracked up.

This time, when Dr. Ackerman entered the room, he introduced me to his nurse Katy, a curly-haired woman in a purple blazer and polka-dotted pants who would be a part of my care team as well. First we would go over my medical history together, Dr. Ackerman told me. Then he would invite my parents in for a conversation about the potential route forward.

"Let's listen to you," he said, placing his hand firmly on my shoulder, looking me in the eyes. "Where does your heart story begin?"

Then, for an hour, he listened, taking careful notes. His eyes—and Katy's—remained on mine, even as he reached backward to pull a box of tissues closer to me. The day in the parking lot. The diagnosis in Utah. The second opinion with Dr. Oza. The long months of waiting. The first surgery. Sepsis. Taking myself off beta-blockers. The accidental shocks. The battery vibration. The clavicular crush. The decision to extract. The wire snap. And the long months of trying to get to Mayo, worrying about politics. Never in my life had someone been so deadly serious in his listening. Never in my life had I been asked, from start to finish, what long QT had been for me. From time to time Dr. Ackerman asked questions, gentle clarifications, but never did he cut me off or offer an early opinion or make it seem like what I had chosen to share was off-topic. And so my heart story stitched itself together.

When we both felt like the story was complete, Dr. Ackerman called a ten-minute break, asking me to retrieve my parents from their seats outside the cardiology entrance, my dad working on his iPad, my mom filling in a crossword puzzle. Dr. Ackerman would record his charting by telephone, he told them as they settled into the exam-room chairs, and we should stop him if we heard anything incorrect in his portrayal.

Then he leaned into the desk, stared at the notes he'd taken, and with the receiver in his hand perfectly repeated back everything he'd heard in my story, everything he knew about our family history, what he'd seen in my dad's and uncle's EKGs. The act was, after so many years, astonishing.

I had been heard.

Dr. Ackerman put the phone down. He turned to us.

"The only wrong things that have been done so far," he said, "are everything that's been done so far."

* * *

The first order of business, Dr. Ackerman said, was to confirm that I actually had long QT syndrome, type 2. The length of my QT on electrocardiograms, the subtle but visible flattening of the contour of my T waves, Christine's genetic results—all this meant I'd likely gotten a correct diagnosis. Because type 2 is known for postpartum-triggered cardiac events, he agreed that it was plausible that Lena Proctor was our missing link—that the defect had come from my dad's side. But given how high the stakes were, Dr. Ackerman recommended mutation-specific genetic testing for all three of us.

I could feel a fantasy opening inside me, one I hungered for: in which I was free of all this because it had all been a mistake, because genetics could tell us conclusively that I'd never had long QT syndrome.

But Dr. Ackerman was moving forward, assuming this would be confirmation and not revelation. If I did have long QT type 2— and I probably did—the question was what level of treatment would adequately protect me. In his kind way, Dr. Ackerman was careful not to ascribe blame to any particular physician. But he also made it clear that we were starting over, reenvisioning my treatment plan from the ground up. He made it clear that he had serious questions about whether I needed an ICD.

I had heard him talk about ICDs in our interview. I picked him as my doctor in part because I believed he was able to realistically see when ICDs were the right tool and when they weren't. Still, it was a breathless thing, a hollow of sudden vulnerability in my stomach, to think of a future in which I was no longer a cyborg. To think it was possible I had been right—that maybe I'd never needed an ICD at all.

"I don't think I should be beholden to another colleague's treatment program," Dr. Ackerman said, "however thoughtfully it was chosen."

One of the biggest questions he had, based on my story, was whether I could have tolerated beta-blockers if I'd been prescribed a lower dose and if they had been more slowly uptitrated. We didn't know, he pointed out, the lowest level of beta-blocker that could provide protection or how I responded to other LQT2-targeted medications. (I didn't know there *were* non-beta-blocker medication options, I told

232

him.) Many people were successfully treated for type 2 long QT with only medications, he said, especially those like me with resting QTs under five hundred milliseconds.

If beta-blockers remained a nonstarter, Dr. Ackerman told me, a growing body of research showed that a procedure called left cardiac sympathetic denervation was providing a significant antifibrillatory protective effect in people with LQT1 and LQT2. "Of course, a denervation procedure doesn't cure long QT," he said, "and it has risks of its own. But these risks are far fewer over the long term than the risks of having an ICD."

Finally, he said, if it looked like we needed to keep some kind of device, we could consider pacing out of the atrial chamber. "Often in type 2, the arrhythmia is set off by a sudden pause in the heart followed by a short coupled skipped beat, which then triggers the substrate into chaos," Dr. Ackerman said. Pacing would keep this from ever happening—rendering defibrillation unnecessary—and it meant fewer and lighter leads in the heart. As a downside, though, they'd likely need to pace at a rate around ninety beats per minute. Some people didn't notice, but someone sensitive to her own body, whose heart rate normally rested much lower—like me—might go a little crazy. "But it could be worth a try," he said, and I agreed.

But we weren't just rebuilding my long QT treatment plan that week; we were also attending to the wire shard in my right ventricle. "In Kati's situation," Ackerman said, "there are a myriad of if-then clauses that we'll need to process through, to determine the best way to proceed."

We wouldn't know until the next day, after my consultation with a surgeon—Dr. Rea—whether extraction of the abandoned lead was deemed possible and necessary. But if we were to attempt a lead extraction in the coming weeks, Dr. Ackerman said, there was a real risk that we might disrupt the functioning leads in my heart. If this happened, we would need to know, roughly, whether we were placing new wires or taking my current ICD out, and if I went without an ICD, I'd need another form of backup.

Here Dr. Ackerman cringed a little. "I can't say I recommend wearing a LifeVest in Tucson during the summer." It was a garment worn beneath the clothes, a full vest with armholes and a back panel that held electrodes against your skin. It had a monitor the size of a paperback book that you wore like a fanny pack. If you were about to be shocked, the electrodes would shoot out a conduction fluid. And you wore this…all the time. Until the medical team felt confident you were protected by another part of your treatment plan.

In order to make a careful decision about removing the ICD, Dr. Ackerman said, we'd need more time. Time to try beta-blockers at low doses, time to try other medications, time to atrially pace or assess the potential of a sympathetic denervation procedure. Time, at a minimum, to get the genetic test results back.

Yet it was time that concerned me, I told him. I'd gotten pre-authorization, but it would expire within a few months. And I had insurance, I told him, but the political landscape made me worry that I wouldn't have any in the future.

"How are you feeling right now?" Dr. Ackerman asked me, as we began to gather our things.

"Overwhelmed," I said. "Confused."

"Overwhelmed and confused is the exact right thing to be feeling as the puzzle pieces fly around our heads," Dr. Ackerman said. "We'll be in touch after your appointment with Dr. Rea tomorrow. In the meantime, here is my business card"—he handed me the square of paper—"and here is Katy's. You can contact us any time with questions. My direct e-mail is listed there."

And then we went out into the rain.

My cardiac surgeon was a wry man with thinning graying hair and rimless glasses who immediately charmed my parents. "Don't take a nap on the park benches in this town," Dr. Robert Rea told us, "or you'll wake up with someone trying to give you CPR."

He'd looked at the X-ray sent by Tucson Medical Center, he said, and he wasn't concerned. He thought the snapped wire could be removed femorally—with a snare and traction, perhaps again using the laser—or maybe from the jugular vein on the right side of my neck, which would allow him to pull at a straighter angle and lessen the effects on my tricuspid valve.

"The reason Mayo is so good is not individual doctors but the systems," he told us humbly—"the excellence of the teams."

The questions at hand, then, revolved around what Dr. Ackerman had called "the myriad if-then clauses." This was June 13. I was scheduled for my surgery on the fifteenth, he said, only the wrong billing code had been used—I was on the schedule for a lead revision in the cardiac cath lab, not an extraction with a cardiac surgery team on standby. We would need to see if the insurance issue could be worked out and if the right facilities were available that day. I'd planned to stay and have surgery that same week, but these factors meant that maybe we shouldn't stay in Rochester—maybe we should go back to Illinois and return when we were booked in the right facility, with the right preauthorization.

The idea of another wait made me itchy. I had this window.

But there were many questions I would need to attend to before I went under, and the answers weren't all obvious. We didn't necessarily need to wait until we had Dr. Ackerman's conclusions about my future long QT treatment in order to go after this broken wire, but, Dr. Rea said, the risks were similar to driving on a highway: if you grouped your trips, you'd travel the route fewer times, with fewer chances for things to go wrong. Medically, it would be helpful if we did the surgery when we knew whether we were taking out my functioning lead wire, too. At a minimum, we would need to know whether we were implanting a new one if the functional lead was disrupted during the procedure. If they couldn't get the broken lead shard femorally or through the jugular, did I want it out come hell or high water? Would I authorize them to cut open my chest? Or should they open my chest only if it was an emergency?

I would also likely have a valve replacement in my future, Dr. Rea said gently, because of damage from the wires. It was an option to wait and do these at the same time, since nothing urgent was happening with the broken lead today.

That kind of wait seemed impossible. Delaying care so strategically was a privilege accessible only to those who knew their ability to access insurance wouldn't shift with the political winds. Even as we sat in that office, the Senate was toying with ways to pass the AHCA, the destructive health-care bill the House of Representatives had already passed, or something similar enough to land them in a reconciliation process. Whenever I mentioned this part of my calculus, Dr. Rea's eyes flashed with concern. It was, of course, not what he would base his medical decisions on. Still, he never belittled or minimized my concerns, and this freed me up to listen more closely to his medical opinion, even if I was still silently running the numbers on how long I had before this set of prior authorizations ran out, whether I thought I could do this again before the end of the year, and how I would support myself if I were living in the contingency of medical procedures.

Dr. Rea reminded me, as he had to, of the risks: stroke, myocardial infarction, pulmonary embolism, cardiac tamponade, bleeding, infection, damage to the normal conduction system of the heart, damage to the valves requiring future repair or surgery, death. And at the end, he suggested one more thing we could do to help clarify the risk of disrupting functional wires: he could send me for a 3-D X-ray the next morning.

"It appears she probably does not need a dual-chamber ICD," my chart would later read. "However, that has yet to be determined. There is no urgent indication to remove the right ventricle lead fragment; however, it has been causing a great deal of anxiety. The longer that fragment stays in her body, the chances of success would go down and the risk of complications would be higher."

I trusted Dr. Rea. I also, listening to him, had found myself full of the sensations of surgery, the places flesh would be cut, the clots that could dislodge, the quiet inner ripping. If I had been unconscious by anesthetic standards for my three procedures, my body itself had been present for all of it—the spitting of the valve, the panic of a circulatory system jerked sideways, the hook in my heart. A man like Dr. Rea, exuding confidence, could make it seem reasonable to undergo these procedures, but they were, in actuality, a wild thing we humans did, a little insane, an expedition into the deeps.

After we left Dr. Rea's office, my parents and I walked west aimlessly, stopping in a grassy park with white stone tables outside one of the medical school buildings. I needed to decide whether we would stay in town, in anticipation of a procedure in a few days, or whether we would turn the car back to Illinois for what could be a short wait or an interminable wait as I wound my way through Dr. Ackerman's recommendations. I had decision fatigue, exhaustion from weighing all the factors and strategizing the route. So much was unknowable. My parents lay on the cool stone benches under the leaf-filtered sunlight and (despite Dr. Rea's instructions) napped. They could help me identify all the factors at play if I wanted them to, but the decisions were mine to make.

I wanted it over. And yet by then I knew that, too often, to solve one problem was to create another. To solve a heart condition with a defibrillator was to bulldoze the jungle. To offset a mine's footprint was to cut off locals from the traditions of their ancestors. To offer a few conservation jobs was to disrupt a community's social ecosystem. I could have lived indefinitely with a capped-off nonfunctional wire inside me, but instead I'd gambled on the procedure, and ended up with this drooping thing in my vena cava.

I could not, I felt, continue to live with the wire inside me. Could not walk back into a future in which this lay ahead, again. But as I strummed my fingers up and down the soft uncut flesh of my breastbone, I was not sure I could tell someone to saw my bones open, to slit the muscle of my heart. I didn't know how a person could become sure about that.

We would wait the week. Dr. Rea would assemble a team. As we drove away from Rochester, a quiet franticness rose in me: as though the Mayo Clinic would not be there when I turned to go back. It was the first place I'd felt safe in a very long time.

At home in my childhood bedroom I made a flowchart for packing. If it was a jugular procedure, I would need loose-necked shirts to accommodate arm-movement restrictions. If it was a femoral procedure, I would need clothing loose at the groin. If it was an open heart procedure, others would need to put me together—and so straps they could pull up, maybe a tube top, a zipper-fronted dress.

On the day before the surgery, we arrived in Rochester again, this time on the Saint Marys campus, where my procedure would occur the next day. My appointment was for a blood draw. Instead, in swept Dr. Rea, fresh out of another procedure, wearing his blue surgical bonnet and scrubs. Something, I knew immediately, was wrong. There would be no blood draw. He leaned forward at the computer, and I stood over his shoulder as he pulled up the X-rays, and zoomed in, and zoomed in, and zoomed in.

There, as expected: three ghostly gray wires, two in the right ventricle and one in the right atrium. Their corkscrew tips, their thick dark defibrillation coils, the slight white line of insulation traveling upward out of the heart. Except for one: the one that ended abruptly, the one that had broken off. This one rose at first from the wall of the heart—a helix and a coil—and then abruptly spidered into three smaller lines, which twisted and curled. A tangle.

I had a nest of wire in my right ventricle, Dr. Rea told me. In Dr. Garrick's tugging a year earlier, the insulation must have been jerked off the semiconductors. The three escaped wires uncoiled themselves in the space of my heart. Over time they grew wild.

He and his team could still try the procedure if I wanted, he told me, concern in his dark brown eyes. But he worried that as he advanced the laser sheath over the nest, the nest would bunch up, a snowplow effect, keeping the sheath from getting as close to the tip as it needed to. And in order to get sufficient traction to unscrew the tip, he would have to tug fairly hard on the spidered wires; without their supporting insulation, he worried they would snap, leaving an even smaller shard embedded in my heart. That the tip of the helix—the corkscrew—was partially retracted from Dr. Garrick's attempt raised the risk of the procedure, making it more likely to tear the muscle.

In the waiting room, my parents looked up in surprise when we entered the room, Dr. Rea in his white coat smiling, extending his hand, ushering them back into the exam room with us, where he repeated the analysis, rubbing his surgical cap between his fingers, adjusting his rimless glasses. My parents staring and staring at the image.

He'd sent the X-rays around, he said, to many of Mayo's top cardiologists. No one recommended the procedure. "The likelihood of complete removal," he said, toying with my chart in its plastic sleeve, "is three in four, one in two." The numbers seemed as though they made him feel a little ill. "When we're doing an infection"—attempting to remove wires from the heart of a person with sepsis—"and the lead starts to fray, that's when it gets tough."

"If it can't be removed through the veins," I said, "this means it can only be removed through open heart surgery?"

"As an open chest procedure, the surgeon would find it very easy, actually," he said. The cut to retrieve the shard would be small and neat. "They might even be able to do it off pump. But it's not causing any problem at the moment in terms of heart function." He looked at me carefully. "That doesn't mean we can't choose to do it, if you want it out come hell or high water. But I will be honest." He rubbed his surgical cap again. "I asked the other doctors. These are some of the most talented cardiac surgeons in the country. They all said, Why the hell would you do that? Cut the sternum of a healthy young person. When the wire isn't causing a problem." The problems, if they occurred, would bloom later: scar tissue buildup, which could affect the heart's conductivity or contraction. If the nest moved around at all, it could affect the functional lead. And, as before, the wires would need to be removed in the case of sepsis.

"So," my mom asked, "when should we expect to remove it?"

At this, Dr. Rea gave a little side smile. "You'll want to take it out," he said, "the day before you have to."

EPILOGUE

Among the Amerindians of the northern Andes, metals were a way of speaking to the gods. A miner or a smith lived as a sort of priest, a creator, a transformer, one working with the gods according to alloy, color, size. It was a gift to find something in the stream that contained such beauty, to see it made into an object of use. Its gleam; the shape of an animal or a bird. Each object was forged of cultural meaning, by technical and magical work, its characteristics fashioned according to the message of the offering. Given as gifts to man, metal objects returned to the earth as gifts to gods in ceremonies high in the mountains, a plea to restore balance in the world.

A defibrillator is an object of cultural meaning. It is an object that holds within it an argument about how we should live and how we should be in the world. That argument is one that prizes expensive electronic technology above other interventions, and it's one that sees death as a failure to be prevented. I do not mean to say that electronic technologies have no place within medicine, but I do mean to say that we live in a system that jumps right to them for reasons of profit and ego and fear: such a technology makes us feel powerful in the face of death, powerful as agents against it. In the story of the defibrillator, the device itself is the hero, the surgeon is the hero—not the patient, living out what it means to be human, which is to say, living out what it means to be subject to death and go on living. I can say firsthand how little our culture is interested in teaching us how to live with death. How different would my story be if we lived in a culture that saw death not as a failure, but as something to dance with? For death is no monolith, and it will not be fixed. Even when we prevent the clinical lifelessness of one body, death comes to us in its gradations, and it will not stop coming, no matter how many technological interventions we offer. I wonder at the story I might have lived if I had been offered, instead of just a slit and a wire, six months of work with a death doula or a trauma-focused mental health practitioner who supported the death-facing young. Or if I'd had access first to a Zoll LifeVest, to slow the decision-making process, allowing time to tweak the medications, while still keeping me safe? So much of my scrambling for a technological solution was an inability to live daily life once diagnosed, in a system that seemed itself unclear whether I was fine or at dire risk.

The defibrillator is also a cultural object in that it is designed to be single-use. Must it be? The first version approved by the FDA was single-use, and so this is the model that's been improved upon, patent by patent. In the context of an economy built around single-use objects, the defibrillator seems normal, and yet there's so much about our medical system and relationship to resource extraction in which "normal" must no longer be acceptable. It is not good enough.

Outside Detroit, a fledgling initiative called My Heart Your Heart is building a replicable process for recycling devices. In five tiny rooms over 450 square feet at the new Sheldon and Marion Davis Pacemaker Recycling World Headquarters, premed students and other volunteers fish used pacemakers out of the industrial gray plastic tubs stacked against the wall—the latest shipments from funeral homes. Each device is checked electrically, and those with at least four years of battery life enter a process of cleaning, interrogation, and sterilization. The devices can't be implanted in the United States because of FDA regulations, but a cardiologist named Dr. Thomas Crawford and his collaborators stash them in their suitcases and fly abroad, to hospitals where local physicians have worked with their governments to approve free implantations. The team placed the first-ever pacemaker in Sierra Leone in 2017—a feat that made it into the news, sixty years after pacing entered clinical practice in the United States.

The team is first recycling pacemakers, rather than defibrillators, because of the increased urgency of the conditions they treat; pacemakers send small, consistent amounts of electricity to a heart to keep it beating, rather than reversing relatively rare cardiac events such as my sister's. Implanted cardiac defibrillators are also more complex devices, with more that can go wrong, requiring a level of sophistication in troubleshooting that may outpace cardiologists at a surgery center where few patients can afford the technology. And pacemakers are ubiquitous, offering a steady supply for recycling, and accumulating into a heap of medical waste if not.

But My Heart Your Heart isn't the only research group working on the problem, and Dr. Behzad B. Pavri of Thomas Jefferson University Hospital, in Philadelphia, has chosen to implant upwards of eighty used ICDs at Holy Family Hospital in Mumbai.

There's no shortage of devices fit to be reimplanted. In addition to devices collected at funeral homes and hospitals, Medicare reimbursement policies consistently send a stream of used devices back to the manufacturers, and warranty-related expiration dates create a pool of legally unusable but essentially brand-new devices. After three years of work, My Heart Your Heart has secured FDA approval to run a series of blind trials that could make implanting used devices abroad more widely accepted. The study will examine whether recycled pacemakers have higher rates of failure than single-use devices—from infections, device malfunctions, or premature battery depletions—or whether their only downside is a slightly reduced battery interval because of the initial use. There's robust disagreement in the cardiology community over whether using recycled devices abroad creates standards of care in low- and middle-income countries that we wouldn't allow in our own hospitals, or whether the offering of a recycled pacemaker should be viewed as saving lives that would otherwise be lost because of a lack of options. A small study of Dr. Pavri's Indian patients published in *Annals of Internal Medicine* suggested no elevated levels of risk, and a full 54 percent of his patients experienced an appropriate shock within the first two years and three months of implantation. That's a more robust rate than in the United States, because only the highest-risk patients at Holy Family Hospital received an ICD.

In a place like Sierra Leone, a new pacemaker costs upwards of $2,000, and ICDs cost several times that—both more than the per-capita GDP. The lead wires alone, at $200 to $300 each, max out what many families can raise. My Heart Your Heart offers the devices at no charge to the patients and estimates that its sterilization and shipping costs—covered by private donations and grants—run just $75 to $100 per device. Yet real challenges remain, since many patients are from rural areas far from a major medical center, making follow-up expensive and complicated.

Beyond sterilization, testing, and reimplantation of a device, the responsible reuse or recycling of the electronic components inside an ICD—rather than their destruction—is the least we can ask for. Yet of the major medical device manufacturers, only Medtronic has initiated a metals recovery program to help dismantle its defibrillators at their end of lives. Meanwhile, this company—and all others in the field, to varying degrees—continues to oppose efforts to reuse devices. They point instead to their own donations of devices as a better option, even though the rate of those dying from lack of access to ICDs—one to two million people annually—far outstrips the rate of their giving. In the United States, those with insurance can access a device they may not actually need, becoming a regular customer of the medical device industry in order to "play it safe" (whether or not it's actually safer than prognosis to implant these devices)—while in the countries more likely to bear our resource burden, those whose lives would be quickly saved have little hope of implantation.

Away is a place. To create a defibrillator and discard it is an act that comes with enormous ecological and social cost. And as my long journey has made clear: all mining takes apart the land, all refining processes carry toxic consequences, and both are destructive to human, animal, and plant life. The only solution I can offer is that we take our rock more carefully. That we remember it as mountain, as sacred object. That if we revere it for saving lives, we allow it to continue doing its work as long as possible and finally decommission it with the care afforded one who has served.

"All men are designers," writes Victor Papanek. "All that we do, almost all the time, is design.... The planning and patterning of any act towards a desired, foreseeable end constitutes the design process." The way we, as individuals, design our days shapes the planet. The way we, as individuals, experience our proximity to death in the midst of a medical crisis shapes the planet, too. If a defibrillator has been designed exhaustively to tackle the *causa finalis* of preventing sudden death and the *causa formalis* of sitting inside the body, directly connected to the heart, with all the impressive technical challenges this entails, its design has never yet taken into account a requirement that it be easily dismantled for reuse of parts, or a requirement that it endure through multiple uses, multiple bodies. Its design has never taken into account that it is earth, that it comes at a cost to other places and people. The prevailing logic of the next defibrillator must include a sense of its future; the manufacturers who act as the *causa efficiens* must engineer a path beyond the single-use object, tossed into an incinerator.

They are not responsible alone. But they are responsible.

"What do you think is a good relationship between business and society?" I'd asked a mining consultant years before in South Africa, on the way home from Madagascar.

"One where it's honest," he said. "Where they trust each other. Where they can work out problems without it escalating to death or production lost." There was no cookie cutter for these things, he explained. They had to be driven by contextual reality. A mining company never had a blank slate. "They're entering history," he said. "And you're going to change the society forever." At a minimum, one should aim to cause no harm, but if it happens, and the company does cause harm, they need to be willing to account for it, clean it up, rectify it. A company couldn't be led, first and foremost, by their budget. They were tenants on others' land. If they hadn't always acted with integrity, he said, the first step was to make it right. The second step was to begin moving dynamically with the community's needs, out of a real trust.

In this framework, a mining company has an ethical obligation to act as a dynamic and vulnerable entity. And yet how can a corporation do that in an era that prizes shareholder gains over everything else? Even when companies claim to have multiple priorities, the word *priority* itself points to singularity. In the moment two priorities clash, one always wins out. The profit mandate takes precedence over delivering health care that is accurate, appropriate, and nourishing; the profit mandate means that a downturn in the metals market leads to inattentiveness to the ways communities' needs are shifting.

Yet I believe in disruptive design: that we can use as our starting point in innovation a demand for what must be, and work backward from there. Those who claim that the current way is the only way are hiding from the work that lies before us all. What would a defibrillator that has its next life built into it look like? Or a model of health care that holds at its center truly *seeing* patients, so that the application of technology is necessary and carefully chosen and so that the important human work of facing death is taken into account? Or a culture of mining that prioritizes community control over extractive projects, rather than profit by outsiders?

We have more power to create something different than we are willing to admit.

The afternoon Dr. Rea told me the wire was a nest, and that it could only be removed by open heart surgery, at some indeterminate point in the future—*the day before you have to*—I left my parents and went up into my hotel room. The Kahler Grand had accidentally booked my parents and me in separate buildings, and as a consolation, they'd upgraded me into a corner room, high in the sky, the kind with two glass walls for looking out over the city, its network of skywalks between hospitals and hotels. I sat in the middle of that very white bed and cried, because it was very possible I had never needed the device, and because now I would never be free of the medical system that made the error. Because so much had happened that was unnecessary, and because now it felt like it was guaranteed to continue. Even if I someday removed the device, we would have to monitor my nest, my trashed valve, for the rest of my life.

On that day, I at least felt like I had the right doctors on my team. I didn't know that I would never make it back to the Mayo Clinic. That I would spend seven months fighting with insurance to get them to pay Mayo for what they'd preauthorized. That in the meantime I would receive giant bills with collection notices. That this would intimidate me from continuing my care, and that the preauthorization would expire. That the only electrophysiologist in-network on my Tucson insurance besides Dr. Garrick would fail to read my records before offering me medical advice, and would sneer at the idea that I needed to go to Mayo. "If you surveyed all electrophysiologists," he said, "how many of them would say you need an ICD? Almost all of them, I bet." To him, this finished the conversation. Once an ICD patient, always an ICD patient.

I would try to go to Mayo as a self-pay patient, having my tests done in-network first and sent over, so that my out-of-pocket costs would be limited to consultation fees: but one test came in a file format Mayo couldn't read and somehow couldn't be converted, and the other tests couldn't be done locally at the level Mayo needed. During a period in which I was earning little money, I would try to go to Mayo on Arizona Medicaid—finally able to access a wider network of physicians, including cardiologists at the university hospital who respected Dr. Ackerman's work and were willing to refer me—only to learn that Mayo didn't accept out-of-state Medicaid patients because the payments were too low to be worth their time. Mayo turned me into a self-pay patient, added a business office appointment to the beginning of my day, and I canceled.

This was not the ending I wanted. When I can, I will have the device removed. I cannot tell you when it will be, or what hijinks will make it possible. I can only tell you I am more afraid of the technology than the genetic mutation. I have come to see metal as sacred enough—and our health-care system as destructive enough—to avoid where I can the manufacturing of a microelectronic. I carry the nest of wire hot inside me: a daily reminder of the death that finds us all.

My best watchman, my worst friend.

* * *

For these questions, there are no final answers. There are only attempts, next steps based on the hard work that lies before us. I see many steps: To prioritize access to health care, so that one's life is affected only by the disease itself, rather than the process of seeking care. To actively train physicians away from their own egos and toward tenderness, understanding what it means to step into the story of a life. To begin the hard cultural work of facing the death that is already around us. To ask that health systems recognize rare conditions and send patients to those most qualified to treat them. To require that the manufacturers of products no longer proceed as though their products will simply disappear—that the next life of any product must honor where it first came from, and what it took to make it. To treat minerals and materials as the sacred substances they are.

In the same way we are "not allowed" to be hysterical within a hyperrational health-care system, we have not been allowed to grieve our mountains. To recognize that we are rummaging inside a body. To see those veins for how they lace into the earth. Might we walk with different humility if we remembered ourselves this way? Brief, made of mineral, and born of earth. Becoming it again.

ACKNOWLEDGMENTS

To my agent, Bonnie Nadell, without whom this book never would have come to be.

To my (very patient) editorial team at Little, Brown Spark, Tracy Behar and Ian Straus—thank you for believing in me and this wild, wild book. To my smoking marketing and publicity team, Jules Horbachevsky, Jessica Chun, and Shannon Hennessey. Carolyn Levin, you set my mind at ease. Barbara Clark, every book should have such a tireless copyeditor.

To Team G.D.—Bethany Nitz-Maile and Jenny O'Connell—you are my Ride or Die, my Hail Mary readers. Your fingerprints are all over this manuscript and I am so grateful.

To Dave Mondy and Tommy Mira y Lopez, for being in it for the long haul. To Merete Mueller in thanks for your sharp eyes and big heart. To Naomi Williams, for lending me your sensitivity, grammar sense, and resilience in the final weeks. To Neda Touloui-Semnani, trauma writing sister, who introduced me to the power of the bathtub.

To the University of Arizona MFA, who gave me my life: I present to you my real thesis, six years late. To Chris Cokinos, my champion and friend, who gifted me Heidegger, took me to my first mine in years, and taught me most of what I know about research. To Ander Monson, who broke open my voice. To Alison Hawthorne Deming, who held space for the struggle between love of land and my life. To all the other writers and faculty in UAMFA, but especially Megan Kimble, who told me early on it was a book, and who taught me how to trust an editor. To Paco Cantú, for kicking my ass into finishing the agenting process, and for answering so many questions over mezcal. To Natalie Lima, for pointing to where my privilege lives on the page. Erin Zwiener, a hundred times you have made me braver. Every writer should have a *Jeopardy!* winner as their copyedits "Phone-a-Friend." Thank you for carrying me the last mile.

To Terry Tempest Williams, for showing me the life I wanted to live upon the land, and what the voice of an artist should be. To Nancy Shea, for reminding me a cell phone is made of mountains. To Chris Bachelder, for your early faith (Skull and Bones forever). To Lisa Jones, whose writing circles opened my way forward. To Jim Miks: always I am trying to be who you knew I was, "one upon whom nothing is wasted." To Bruce Janu, for holding the intellectual space I so needed as a young person. With love to my original Writer's Circle at John Hersey High School, and to the English Department circa 2003. (Thanks for giving me the Writing Award even though I never took AP.)

To Whig Mullins and my instructors at Trails Wilderness School, for bringing me to the Wyoming Range, and for teaching me how to read the land. To the First United Methodist Church of Arlington Heights, my truest community, who taught me how to embody empathy. With enormous thanks to the old Murie Center in Moose, Wyoming, with its legacy of conservation writers: both land and people formed me as a thinker. That riverbend, those forests are still my most sacred place.

Thanks to the Sociology and English departments at the Colorado College, especially professors Gail Murphy-Geiss, Jeff Livesay, Maria Varela, Wade Roberts, Eric Popkin, Regula Evitt, and Teresa Cohn, for showing me how to move through the world asking questions. The Colorado College Award in Literature taught me, way back at the beginning, how to write a book.

To Arthur Frank, whose book *The Wounded Storyteller* guided me back to my life.

To Zhenevere Sophia Dao, for a lifetime of calling me to beautiful risk.

ACKNOWLEDGMENTS

I'm endlessly grateful for those who supported the book in its early years, when the concept seemed unfeasible. The University of Arizona Writing Program's 2013 Writing Fellowship gave me room to find my mine and write through the first major arc of the memoir.

Thanks to the nearly three hundred supporters of the 2014 Kickstarter Project that funded research in Madagascar and South Africa, including but not limited to Taylor Lenton, Molly Armour, Kenneth Maltas, Shannon Hogan, Judy Craver, Kyle Marquette, Sarah McKellar, Shannon Lange, Jan Abramczyk, Kristine Bentz, Jonathan Chiou, Andrew Perkins, Megan Leith, Cathy Dombi, Kendra Murray, Theresa Stein, Cedes Hoffman, Lauren Watel, Kathy O'Dowd, Melissa Slocum, Svetlana Kurakina, Jeff Zwiener, Archimedes Gordon, Fyetka Gordon, Finneas Gordon, Iryna and Matt Marchiano, Larry Fuschino, Chris Benz, and Laura Parker. In memoriam to my special patron, the inimitable Marian "Joso" Souder.

Thanks to the fifty-one souls who contributed to medical bills and additional research funding in the summer of 2016 via GoFundMe. Thanks to the 121 hearts who helped keep me afloat through GoFundMe in the summer of 2017, as I fought to get to Mayo and then grieved. Thanks to Team Awesome—Martyna Skura and Swiff Lui—who got me through the first broken wire summer in Arusha with love and Konyagi. *Iko moja*. Thanks to my coworkers and students in Costa Rica, who tenderly helped me live my way into what came next.

Thanks to all who support my work monthly via Patreon, but especially: Briana Aragon, Charlie Buck, Christine Barbetta, Jared Spaulding, London Vallery, Eva Chartier, CRC Montgomery, Danielle Ezzo, Wendy Fox, Eric LeMay, Frederic Lange, Jen Gilman-Porat, Paula Marchiano, Leslie Pollack, Lauren Zeppo, and Pat Dolan.

Thank you to Bruce and Creigh Day, for never in seven years raising my Tucson rent.

Thanks to the Mesa Refuge for hosting my frenzied book proposal writing, supported by Marion Weber and her Healing Arts Fellowship. Essential portions of this book were written at the Centre d'Art i Natura in Farrera, Catalonia, Spain, and the Jentel Foundation in Banner, Wyoming, both of which gave me back my soul. I'm eternally grateful to the Jonathan Logan Family Foundation for the opportunity

ACKNOWLEDGMENTS

to work alongside my brilliant cohort in the Logan Nonfiction Fellowship Program at the Carey Institute for Global Good. (Sorry about the Ebola.) Much thanks to Kaospilot and the Unschool, especially Andy Sontag and Emma Segal, for their #PostDisposable program in Aarhus, Denmark, which allowed me to envision how we might ask more of our corporations, using design to intentionally reshape our world. I'm cowed by the fellowship and support of the Ashland University low-residency MFA faculty and community; thank you to Christian Kiefer for that gift of a lifetime.

Portions of this book appeared in altered form in *The Colorado Review, The Normal School, Terrain,* and *Kenyon Review Online.* I'm especially grateful to Stephanie G'Schwind for her early faith, and to Simmons Buntin for his cyborgy friendship.

To Chelsea Biondolillo, for reminding me of the stories I held when the book seemed impossible.

To Sarah Estill, for bringing a pot to my empty Boulder apartment, for bringing a casserole to my hospital room, for showing up for me and my writing repeatedly, in ways I didn't even know I needed.

To Kali and Sonja on Glorieta Mesa: your Earth Home allowed me to write what I thought was stuck in me forever. To Maddie Norris, in gratitude for the stunning gift of your home when I had nowhere to land. To Deb and John Kuzloski, who allowed me to come home to Wyoming again and again. To Raymond Ansotegui and Amber Jean, for stringing an extension cord up a mountain. To Mike and Amber Hoover, for the magic of a cabin in Kelly, finally sleeping across from the Grand again.

More than anywhere else, Exo Roast Company in Tucson, Arizona, held the space of my dreams for the duration of this book project. Thank you to Amy and Doug Smith, Chris Byrne, and all my daily baristas over the years (but especially Adam Stratman): for every ounce of beauty and community, mezcal and Americano. You were my home when I literally didn't have one.

David Zugerman and Jessie Mance, I couldn't have sold this book (or survived those years) without your kindness and grace. Bartending at Tucson Hop Shop was one of the great and unexpected pleasures of my career. #HopShopMyHeart!

ACKNOWLEDGMENTS

Tucson's literary community is richer and fiercer than a town that size could hope for, and there are more of you than I can name. Thank you for inspiring me and celebrating with me. We'll reschedule the party for when every one of you is allowed into the same room.

Danielle Watters, your faith in me opened one of the great pivots of my life. To Bridgett Royer, who once said, "I just assume you'll slip through at the last minute, because that's what Kati Standefer always does." Thank you for reminding me who I am. To Ellen Teig, for never doubting this book would come to be. Dear PJ, who swooped in to save me: thank you for calling her Nurse Ratched. To Kelly Pollard, who I'm still learning from. And to the rest of that staff and community: to serve through Boulder Valley Women's Health Center was the privilege of a lifetime.

To Will Sarni, for hiring me at a pivotal moment and requiring me to read my first corporate social and environmental responsibility reports. Who knew what that would become?

I reported an iceberg of material to offer just the tip. Thanks to all who spoke on and off the record to make sure I understood the landscape of mining, the politics of Madagascar, the unfolding story of corporate social responsibility and conflict minerals legislation, the specifics of conservation efforts, and much more. Thanks to the many health care writers whose work forms the invisible foundation of my own. Thank you Kirk Jeffery, for generously fielding my questions about pacemakers and defibrillators. Thank you to Ed Cooper, for writing our family history, and to Kay Overton and the community of Hamilton, Texas, for showing me where it all unfolded. To Hilary Gan and Brad Kemph, the best L.A. hosts. To Alex and Dave Davis, for drawing the map. Emily Biester, Loren Diesi, and the other Madagascar Peace Corps volunteers of 2014, you are my heroes. I owe such a debt to Marcia and George at Centre Lambahoany. I bow to all my interpreters and guides. Thanks to Devin Edmonds and Maya Moore, for answering questions over the years. To Cathy at the front desk of Hotel Talinjoo, who kept me safe, and all the expats on the porch and at local NGOs, who pointed me in important directions. To Mergan and Sally Govender, for gracious hosting in Johannesburg. To Marcia Male, the best host and happy hour partner imaginable in

Rwanda. To Alvin at the INZU Lodge in Gisenyi, for going down the mine shaft. To Innocent Nkurunziza and the other Inema artists, for showing me the vibrance of your beautiful country. To Kelly Shaw, for a guest bedroom in Minneapolis and driving me to SJM on that rainy morning. To my trainers at Guardian-srm, for making risk mitigation muscle memory. To Dr. Thomas Crawford and Project My Heart Your Heart: I'm so grateful for your work. To the Sudden Arrhythmia Death Syndromes Foundation: thank you for being there to answer my questions, and for your ongoing advocacy for our families. To those in the ICD, S-ICD, and Sudden Cardiac Death Facebook groups who helped me understand my story by sharing their own: thank you.

This book exists as an artifact of my own white privilege and settler-colonial lineage. It was written on the occupied lands of many indigenous people, but especially that of the Tohono O'odham of present-day Arizona, the Shoshone and Cheyenne of present-day Wyoming, and the Pueblo tribes of present-day New Mexico. The book was sold in a structural environment that privileges white writers, and the book's research funding relied in large part on my networks of privilege. A portion of proceeds from this book and its publicity activities will fund acts of reparation. I bow to the Malagasy, Rwandans, and Congolese who invited me into the stories of their homes, despite centuries of exploitation by white-skinned strangers from the West.

To Chrissy Tolley: because every writer needs a psychic. Thank you for calling me back to myself a hundred times, and for getting your hands dirty in the minutiae of my manuscript. To Josh Whiteley, my healer across so many wild years. To Dr. Eric Vindiola, for undoing the damage of the writing desk. To Lindsey Bishop and Grant Freeman, who woke me up. To Lyn Dalebout, who first told me my work this lifetime would be the body. To Lady Bash Quesenberry, for helping me step into my power. To Katherine Gerardi, for transforming how I move through this world. To Lynne MacNeil, who taught me I wasn't crazy, and who made the book physically possible. To Eve Bradford, for casting light on my next tender steps. I have been blessed by more healers than I can name here; you know who you are.

To Mike Shum, for your behind-the-scenes support. I'm both sorry and glad to be in the club. To Hope and Les Law, for teaching me how to move through Africa with grace. To Sarah Diefendorf: let's brag about each other forever. To Chris Benz, for asking me if I was writing in the years I wasn't. To Lauren Markham, worthy of a sacred journalistic trust.

To my oldest friends, who held my writing dream with me from the beginning: Julie Hanson, Kate Kuehn, Emily Labbe Gennaro, Nisha Graves.

To Mary Stitt, my lifelong mentor in global citizenship.

To Liza Sparks, brave poet, who helped keep my soul afloat in the fall of 2009. Could either of us have imagined, sitting there in Trident and the Rocky Flats Lounge, that I was writing passages for my future book? (Maybe yes.)

Thank you to every one of my clients and students: you made me braver.

To Janelle Marchiano Robinson, for formative porch chats, Wednesday morning breakfasts, and Team Vulture. Thank you for inviting your community and family into the circle of my work. And, with Chad Robinson, for literally helping me get to where I needed to go.

To Aaron Chambers: for never letting me die without getting laid first.

To Tiffany Englander: for never doubting my art-making, for always arriving with a letter. Your art is next.

To Dr. Sameer Oza, for your fierce care of our lives.

To Dr. Todd Turner, for seeing me.

To Dr. Michael Ackerman, who healed me first by listening.

To Dr. Robert Rea, the first and only surgeon to call a billing office on my behalf.

To Tony "Julien" Colella, who made it all seem possible from the beginning.

To Sara Hubbs and Lee Anne Gallaway-Mitchell: my book doulas.

To Makendra Silverman: this book is as much yours as mine. Thank you for literally keeping me alive, especially at Red Wing. Your friendship is one of the great gifts of my life. And to Chad Gordon, from one writer to another, for becoming family.

To Becca Reynolds, for laughing with me through everything that is not funny. For being able to hold it when no one else could bear to. I love you always.

To Cindy Standefer Smiskol and Steve and Nancy Eich, for showing up every time I asked, and for taking care of so many people I care about. You are a beautiful presence in my life. To Dave, Sands, and Emma Standefer, who I could feel standing behind me. With thanks to Steve Standefer for his historical assistance and cheerleading; with love to Chris Standefer, part of Team LQT.

It is a source of grief that the Big Shipoopi—Grandpa Bob Eich—did not live to see me publish a book. His estate funded some of my reseach. His spirit remained with me every step.

My dear friend Lois Anderson wanted so badly to read this manuscript. Lois, I'm sorry I took so long. (And: I promise, still and always.)

To Melisa Doran Cole and Tria Aronow, my Three of Cups in this world, who made space for the version of me that needed to be born in order for this book to finish.

To the Tucson climbing crew, who have caught me in every sense of the word: Luke Parsons, the purest kind of friend. Jessica Stahl, who taught me how a heart works. Gloria Jimenez, who believed in me more than me. Diane Thompson, for sunset walks and whiskies. Alison Miller and Nick Henscheid, who took me in and made me family. Kat Compton, who somehow has room for every part of me. From fireside readings to Kickstarter hustling, you all walked with me the whole way.

To "Sam": I know it wasn't the story you wanted. But it was the story I lived. I forgave you a long time ago, and I miss your friendship. Please know: your belief in my writing made it happen.

To my dad, who steeped me in good writing, taught me life was for big journeys, and made it possible to be who I was born to be. (I made it to the place the pavement ends!) You have been brave and kind through so much, and make my heart so tender. Thank you.

To my mom, the real hero of this story. Thank you for always handing me back my key.

And to Christine, who gave me the gift of a lifetime in allowing me to tell her story. Whose life was always worth it. I'm so glad neither of us had to do this alone.

INDEX

Ackerman, Michael, 213, 247
  community presentation by,
    213–15
  narrative medicine interview
    with, 216–17, 218
  treatment plan of, 230–34,
    235, 237
acupuncture, 138, 144
adrenaline spikes, 24, 59,
    137–38
Affordable Care Act
  Medicaid expansion and,
    165, 219
  passage of, 134–35
  premium increases and, 211
  repealing and replacing, 205,
    210–11, 218–19
  subsidies of, 212, 218
Africa
  cardiac care in, 153–54
  mining in South, 70,
    165–67, 245

  summer job in Tanzania,
    164, 169, 186, 199,
    206–8
  See also Democratic Repub-
    lic of the Congo;
    Madagascar; Rwanda
Al Qaeda, 198
Al-Shabaab, 208
Ambatovy mining project
    (Madagascar), 67–68
  agricultural projects of, 93
  Ambohinierenana village
    and, 84
  Ampitambe village and,
    81–83
  Andasibe village and, 85–87
  animal salvaging by, 68–69
  Berapaka village and,
    94–96
  conservation offset by, 88,
    89, 96
  Fetraomby village and, 90

Ambatovy mining project
(Madagascar) (*cont.*)
Maroseranana community
and, 89–94, 96
Moramanga boomtown and,
78–81, 85
Ore Preparation Plant of, 68, 76
preparations to visit, 147
refinery of, 72
social responsibility program
of, 71–73, 80, 82
Toamasina refinery of, 76–77
Vohitranivona village and,
83–84, 85
American Health Care Act,
210–11, 218, 235–36
Americans with Disabilities
Act, 211
ammonium sulfate, 67
Andasibe-Mantadia National Park
(Madagascar), 69, 85–87
Andrew Lees Trust, 159
Apple products, 74–75
arrhythmia
cardiac arrest and, 5–6, 8
heart block, 178
long QT interval and, 21, 30
torsades de pointes, 27, 29,
30, 35, 135, 139, 170
ventricular fibrillation, 35
See also long QT syndrome
Austin, Stephen, 169

bacteremia, 116, 129
Barrick Gold Corporation (Papua
New Guinea), 69–70

Batu Hijau mine (Indonesia), 70
Becker, Ernest, ix
beta-blockers, 11
arrhythmia with, 139
dosage changes in, 29, 55,
232–33, 234
"forgetting" to take, 63
overdose of, 56
side effects of, 25, 26–27,
31, 59, 106
starting on, 22, 23, 24
transitioning off, 137,
138–39, 140–41
zombies created by, 217
birth defects, mining-
associated, 150, 151, 152,
154, 204
blood clots
embolism and, 119–23, 132
femoral artery, 188–89, 190,
191, 195
healing process and, 124–25
postoperative risk for, 220
body
changes in, 111, 117–18
control over, 224
silence from, 97, 132
suffering in, 97, 106
vitality of, 145
Boston Scientific, 177, 184, 216
Boulder Community Hospital
(CO)
infection rate in, 121
sepsis treatment in, 115–18,
120–25
surgery at, 29, 187–94

Burns, Ken, 124
Bush administration, drilling policy of, 78

Camus, Albert, *The Myth of Sisyphus*, 222
cardiac arrest
    arrhythmia causing, 5–6, 8
    faking, 63–64
    heart attack *vs.*, 13
    long QT syndrome and, 10
    prevention of, 216
cardiac tamponade, 182
cardioverter defibrillator, implanted. *See* ICD
cassiterite, 196
cell phones, 74–75, 196
chaos narrative, 224
Chardack, William, 179
chest pain
    heart attack and, 12–13
    long QT syndrome and, 12, 65
    sepsis and, 119, 121, 122, 132
chest tubes, 220
climate change, 89
cobalt
    mining, 67–68, 88
    refining, 72, 77–78
Cole, Melisa Doran, 163, 174
Colella, Tony "Julien," 136, 139, 140
Colorado Indigent Care Program, 33, 63
coltan. *See* tantalum
Compton, Kat, 191–92

Cooperative COMINYABU mine (Busoro, Rwanda), 199–200, 201, 202–203
copper mining, 69, 70
Coumadin, 122–23, 124, 125, 132
Crawford, Thomas, 242
CT (computed tomography) scan, 114
    with contrast, 115, 120–21
    after embolism, 132

Dalrymple, Andra, 213
death
    Becker on, ix
    choosing life over, 207–8, 221–22
    from defibrillator shocks, 141–43
    inevitability of, 241–42, 247
    lack of health care and, 52, 244
    living with, 123, 206, 229, 245
    longing for, 56–57, 61, 224
    long QT syndrome and, 25, 216
    owl sighting and, 187
    sepsis and, 129–30
    stalking by, 26, 217
defibrillators
    battery of, 41, 43, 163, 164, 168, 173–76
    capacitor of, 41, 43, 46, 142
    causa for, 42–43, 224, 245
    as cultural object, 241–42

defibrillators (*cont.*)
ecological and social cost of, 91, 160, 204, 244–45
external and wearable, 184, 233–34, 242
first single-use, 242
Grandma Test for, 45
lack of access to, 244
manufacturers of, 38, 40–48, 177, 184, 216
metals in, 2, 38–40, 41, 68, 179, 244
microelectronics in, 41, 43, 44–45, 68, 75
as miracle device *vs.* tool, 204
pacemakers *vs.*, 153
problems with, 45, 177, 217
recycling, 243–44, 245
thanks owed by, 42, 47
See also ICDs
democracy, natural resources and, 96
Democratic Republic of the Congo (DRC)
conflict minerals from, 39, 40
economic decline in, 73
mining controlled by, 196–99, 201
violence in, 39, 197, 199
diamond mining
in South Africa, 165
wars fueled by, 39–40, 198
Dodd-Frank Act of 2010, 197–98, 199
Dougherty, Cynthia M., 143
Dutch disease, 82

EKG (electrocardiogram), 10
after defibrillator shocks, 135
for family members, 12
invention of, 169
for long QT diagnosis, 20, 21, 30, 232
postoperative, 100
for sepsis, 117
for wire removal surgery, 230
embolism
pulmonary, 119–23, 132
risks for, 125
See also blood clots
Equator Principles, 72, 89

FDA (Food and Drug Administration)
defibrillator approvals by, 47, 179, 184, 242
device recalls by, 177, 180
device recycling regulations of, 242, 243
femoral artery, surgical incision in, 188, 192
clotting of, 188–89, 190, 191, 195
invention of, 205
Flake, Jeff, 210–12
Forest Trends, Business and Biodiversity Offsets Programme of, 71, 88
Frank, Arthur, 164, 193, 224
Furman, Seymour, 178

Garrick, Dr., wire removal
     surgery by, 188, 192–94,
     206, 213, 238
   consultation with, 183–84,
        185, 205, 208, 217–18
   fee for, 212
   insurance authorization for,
        222, 228, 229, 247
   long QT conference and,
        215
   scheduling, 209–10
genetic testing, 232, 234
Global Reporting Initiative
     (GRI), 71
gold mining, 196
   in Arizona, 69
   in Democratic Republic of
        the Congo, 39
   panning in, 93
   in Papua New Guinea, 69–
        70
   regulation of, 197–98
   in South Africa, 165
Grasberg copper mine (Indo-
     nesia), 70
Grateful Dead, 18
Great Recession of 2008, 17,
     20, 33, 197
Grijalva, Raúl, 211

Harken, Dwight, 186
health care
   care vs. profit in, 223–24,
        247
   clinic job in, 104–6, 111–14,
        127, 132, 135, 138

   debates over, 19, 26, 52,
        210–11, 235–36
   health outcomes of, 144–45
   Wyoming and, 33
   See also Affordable Care Act;
        American Health Care
        Act
health insurance
   access to, 32, 235, 248
   catastrophic, 20
   for defibrillator replacement,
        164, 165
   high-risk pools for, 31
   lack of, 20, 29, 52, 205, 209,
        219
   negotiated-down rates for,
        32
   parents' plan for, 19–20
   preexisting conditions in, 19,
        114, 134
   provider options in, 190–91,
        205
   student policy for, 143–44
   waiting period for, 114
   for wire removal, 213, 217–
        18, 222–23, 228, 229,
        235, 247
heart
   blood flow through, 9–10
   contractions of, 177–78
   electrical pulses in, 9–10,
        13, 27, 169, 178
   inflammation and scarring
        of, 117
   open surgery of, 182, 219,
        239, 246

heart (*cont.*)
    sympathetic denervation of,
        233, 234
    tamponade of, 182
    valve replacement in, 235
    ventricular septal defects of,
        178
heart attack, 12–13
heart rate
    beta-blockers and, 11, 25,
        26, 137
    defibrillator and, 100,
        141–42
    See also pacemakers
Heidegger, Martin, "The Ques-
        tion Concerning
        Technology," xiii, 41–42, 87
helium, 41, 48
heparin, 117, 122, 125, 126
HIV, mining town outbreaks of,
        72, 80
Holy Family Hospital (Mum-
        bai, India), 243–44
homelessness, 49–50, 56

ICDs (implanted cardioverter
        defibrillators), 11
    in Africa, 153–54
    bacterial colonization on,
        116, 117, 129, 183
    beta-blockers and, 139
    check-ups of, 100, 132–33,
        137, 140–41, 143–44,
        145
    Christine's, 1, 11–12, 13–14,
        21, 34–35, 37, 45,

        101–2, 132–33, 139–
        40, 164, 174, 185
    disposal of used, 175–76,
        200–201
    Ellipse model of, 45–46
    feelings about, 27–28, 29,
        34, 55, 66, 123
    first implantable, 179
    first surgery for, 30, 31–35,
        62–66, 97–100, 105,
        133–34
    holding in place, 97–98, 106
    lead wires for, 176–81, 200,
        209, 238
    magnets over, 136, 137, 143, 144
    movement restriction from, 99
    need for, 22, 23, 24, 27, 216,
        232, 236, 246, 247
    origin of contents of, 38–41,
        70–71, 196
    removal of, 233–34, 247
    second surgery for, 163–65,
        168–69, 173–76, 181,
        183, 186
    sharing personal story about,
        212
    shocks from, 1–2, 13–14,
        38, 45, 131–32, 135–
        36, 141–43, 145, 196
    silence of, 134, 137, 185
    subcutaneous, 184–86, 217
    third, 176, 200
    twiddler and reel syndromes
        related to, 99
    See also defibrillators; wire
        extraction surgery

ilmenite
    export of, 146
    mining and extraction of,
        148, 151, 155–56, 159
    See also titanium
Industrial Revolution, 82
International Finance Corpora-
    tion, 77
International Tin Supply Chain
    Initiative (iTSCi), 199, 203
iridium, 179

Jackson Hole Center for the
    Arts (WY), 18
Jeffrey, Kirk, 177, 179

Kabila, Joseph, 197, 199
Kimberly Process (United
    Nations General Assem-
    bly), 198

lemurs
    bridges for, 68, 204
    refuge for, 86–87
    tiny stuffed, 98
Liberia, economic decline in, 73
LifeVest, 184, 233–34, 242
lightning flowers, 2, 141
Lillehei, C. Walton, 178
long QT syndrome, 10–11
    Ackerman's philosophy of,
        216
    adrenaline spikes and,
        137–38
    Christine and, 9, 20, 169
    conference on, 213–15

diagnosis of, 13, 20, 21
exercise and, 11, 23, 29, 59,
    141–42
family history of, 12–13, 29,
    169, 173, 232
genetic testing for, 232
lethality of, 25, 216
medication-induced, 10
prevalence of, 25, 214
repolarization time in, 10, 27
sleep and, 11, 26, 35
symptoms of, 12, 18–19, 21,
    26, 65, 169
treatment options for, 27–28,
    232–33, 234
triggers for, 24–26

MacIntyre, Alasdair, ix
Madagascar
    economic inequality in,
        73–74, 82, 95–96, 158
    endemic and endangered
        species in, 67, 72, 73,
        74, 89, 96, 155, 156
    future of communities in, 167
    government of, 147–48, 150,
        158
    health inequity in, 153, 154
    population growth in, 89
    resource extraction in, 74,
        168
    shipping ports in, 146–47
    See also Ambatovy mining
        project; QIT Madagas-
        car Minerals;
        rainforest, Madagascar

magnets
    defibrillator inactivation by,
        136, 137, 143, 144
    mineral separation with,
        151, 155
Mai-Mai militias, 197
malaria, 151–52
Marikana platinum mine
        (South Africa), 70
massage therapy, 138
Mayo Clinic, 213, 216, 227
    billing policy of, 228, 247
    scheduling appointments at,
        217–18, 224–25,
        228
    tests at, 229, 230
    wire removal surgery at,
        230–34, 235, 237–38
Medicaid
    expansion of, 31, 165, 219
    Mayo Clinic and, 247
Medicare
    device recycling and, 243
    surgery reimbursement by,
        179
meditation, 138
Medtronic, 216
    lead wires of, 177, 180
    metal recovery program of,
        244
Meier, Barry, 177, 180
mercury poisoning, 70
metals and minerals
    certified conflict free, 196,
        198–99
    conflict, 39–40, 69, 196

in defibrillator, 2, 38–40, 41,
        68, 179, 244
    DRC conflict undetermin-
        able, 198
    regulation of, 197–98, 199, 203
    sacredness of, 241, 247, 248
Miller, Alison, 191–92
mining, 2
    of conflict minerals, 39–40
    ecological and social cost of,
        69–70, 71, 87, 96,
        167–68, 204, 244–45
    ethical obligations of,
        245–46
    financing of, 72
    in Fort Dauphin, 146–47,
        148–49
    fracking in, 78
    in Indonesia, 70
    protests against, 72, 147–48
    in Questa, NM, 28
    radioactive tailings from,
        159–60, 167
    in Rwanda, 196–203, 206
    in South Africa, 70, 165–67,
        245
    technological advancements
        in, 81–82
    in Uganda, 196–98
    village resettlement in, 67,
        68, 73, 76–77
    in West Texas, 169
    in Wyoming, 28, 69, 78, 167
    See also Ambatovy mining
        project; QIT Madagas-
        car Minerals

miscarriage, mining-associated, 150, 151
Missouri Botanical Garden, 155
molybdenum mining, 28
morphine, 120, 121
My Heart Your Heart, 242–44

natural gas fields
    in West Texas, 169
    in Wyoming, 28, 78
Ndriamiary, Jean-Noël, 87
nervous system, restrengthening, 138, 144
nickel
    mining, 67–68, 88
    refining, 72, 77–78

Obama, Barack, 52, 205
Obamacare. *See* Affordable Care Act
organic solvents, 77
Overton, Kay, 170–72
Oza, Sameer, 52, 141, 231
    beta-blocker prescribed by, 55
    Christine's care by, 6, 8, 11, 13
    fee donation by, 29, 33, 97, 105
    ICD implantation by, 32–33, 62–63, 65–66
    records review by, 29–30
    sepsis evaluation and, 116, 121, 183
    treatment plan of, 27, 29, 30, 106

wire removal surgery and, 208–9
Ozius Spatial, 160

pacemakers
    advancements in, 178–79
    in Africa, 153
    defibrillators *vs.*, 153
    disposal of used, 200–201
    for long QT syndrome, 233, 234
    protester with, 211–12
    recycling, 242–44
    sinus node as, 9
paint, titanium in, 148, 154
Pan-African Society of Cardiology, 153
Papanek, Victor, 245
Pavri, Behzad B., 243–44
PICC (peripherally inserted central catheter), 118–19, 126, 133
platinum
    mining, 70, 165, 166
    in pacemaker lead, 179
pneumonia, 117, 118, 120, 124–25
pollution, mining-related, 150, 159–60
Providencia, Rui, 180

QIT Madagascar Minerals (QMM), 148
    environmental policy for, 159–60
    forest rehabilitation by, 158

QIT Madagascar Minerals
   (QMM) (*cont.*)
   Fort Dauphin and, 148–49
   health problems associated
      with, 150–52
   Mandena Conservation Zone
      of, 149, 155, 156–58,
      159–60
   Mandromondromotra and,
      149–51
   mining process of, 155–56
   Nahampoana village and,
      149, 157
   owners of, 148, 159
   protests against, 148
   tour of, 154
QT interval, long *vs.* normal,
   10, 21, 27, 30
   See also long QT syndrome
Questa molybdenum mine
   (NM), 28

rainforest, Madagascar
   Ankerana, 69, 88–89, 93
   conservation zones in, 69,
      83, 88, 93, 96
   destruction of, 67, 69,
      88–89, 158, 204
   Mandena, 149, 155,
      156–58, 159–60
   mitigation hierarchy for,
      71–72, 88
   reclamation of, 73, 74, 159, 160
   secondary *vs.* littoral, 154–55
Rattlesnake Hills (WY), gold
   mining in, 69

Rea, Robert, 233, 234–36, 237,
   238, 246
Rio Tinto, 148, 152, 159–60
Robinson, Janelle Marchiano,
   219–20
Rocephin, 118
Roe v. Wade, 104
Rwanda
   genocide in, 197, 202
   mining in, 196–203, 206

SADS (Sudden Arrhythmia
   Death Syndromes Foun-
   dation), 24, 25, 75–76,
   213
Sam (boyfriend), 15–17
   Beating Heart Bear surgery
      by, 60–61
   biking and hiking with,
      30–31
   Boulder visits by, 57–58,
      59–60, 62, 64
   breaking up with, 16,
      127–29
   Cape Cod visit with, 102–3
   climbing trip of, 100–101
   cousins of, 29–30, 64
   disconnection from, 53–54,
      105–7, 126–27
   last good day with, 104, 107,
      109–10
   love of, 130
   picnic with, 119–20
   rent checks from, 133
   sailing and camping with,
      35–36

support from, 18–20, 22,
    26–27, 30, 55, 61, 65,
    98, 108–9, 112–17,
    125–26
writing work of, 17, 59–60,
    105
sepsis, 116
    appetite and, 191–92
    blood clot in, 119–23,
        124–25, 132
    copays after, 133–34
    diagnostic tests for, 113–16
    fear of, 183, 195
    Group B streptococcus and,
        129–30
    home care for, 118–19,
        125–26
    hospitalization for, 115–18,
        120–25
    symptoms of, 108–9, 111,
        112–13, 114
    treatment plan for, 145
sex workers and sex slaves,
    79–80, 149, 197, 204
Sheldon and Marion Davis
    Pacemaker Recycling
    Center, 242
Sierra Leone
    blood diamonds from, 39–40
    cardiac devices in, 242–43,
        244
Silverman, Makendra, 54,
    229–30
Silverstein, Shel, *A Light in the
    Attic,* 122, 124
solvents, organic, 77

South Africa, mining in, 70,
    165–67, 245
spinal tap, 114
Standefer, Bertha (wife of
    Henry Standefer), 171,
    172
Standefer, Cecil (great-
    grandfather), 170, 173
Standefer, Christine (sister)
    beta-blockers and, 138–39
    birthday celebrations with,
        73, 228
    body piercing with, 61–62
    cardiac arrest in, 5–6, 8, 26
    defibrillator of, 1, 11–12,
        13–14, 21, 34–35, 37,
        45, 101–2, 132–33,
        139–40, 164, 174, 185
    emotional support from, 37,
        98, 101, 229
    genetic testing of, 232
    living with, 49
    long QT syndrome in, 9, 20,
        169
    relationship with, 9, 101–2
Standefer, David (great-great
    half uncle), 171–72
Standefer, Henry (great-great
    grandfather), 170–71,
    172, 173
Standefer, Katherine E.
    ancestors of, 13, 82–83,
        169–73
    bartending job of, 208, 218
    birthdays of, 86, 127, 228
    bluegrass band with, 16, 18

Standefer, Katherine E. (*cont.*)
  Boulder residency of, 34, 49,
      50–52, 54, 57, 101,
      229
  Broken Arrow Ranch and, 6, 8
  childhood home of, 6–7
  college education of, 7, 19,
      78, 134–35, 138
  female friends of, 54, 163,
      174, 191–92, 201–2,
      219–20, 229–30
  figure modeling by, 33, 65
  global leadership program
      and, 164, 169, 186,
      199, 206–8
  hiking guide job of, 25–26
  job hunting by, 31, 34, 49–
      50, 53
  law firm position for, 58–59,
      61, 62
  parental support of, 12, 19,
      30–34, 50–52, 98,
      99–100, 116, 117–18,
      121–22, 124, 133–34,
      174–75, 181, 187,
      191–92, 236–37,
      238–39
  puzzle factory job of, 104
  research assistant job of,
      105, 133
  sexual health clinic work of,
      104–6, 111–14, 127,
      132, 135, 138
  sisters of, 9, 12, 228. *See also*
      Christine
  ski and rock climbing in-
      struction by, 8, 12, 21
  soccer playing by, 1, 136–37,
      139, 142
  teaching job of, 213, 214
  University Inn and, 52–53,
      54–55
  writing by, 7, 8, 32, 208,
      213–14
Standefer, Lena Proctor (great-
      great-grandmother), 13,
      169–73, 232
St. John's Medical Center
      (Jackson, WY)
  diagnostic evaluation in,
      20–22, 29, 30
  financial aid from, 31
St. Jude Medical, 216
  defibrillator checks by, 100
  defibrillator donation by,
      97
  lead wires of, 177, 180, 181
  patient hotline of, 38–39
  Scottsdale (AZ) facility of,
      43, 44–45
  Sylmar (CA) factory of, 38,
      40–41, 42–48
  used devices returned to,
      200
streptococcus, Group B, 129
stress management, 11, 138
Sudden Arrhythmia Death Syn-
      dromes Foundation (SADS),
      24, 25, 75–76, 213
suicide
  defibrillator shocks and, 143
  ideation of, 56–57, 61

tantalum
    mining, 39, 196, 202
    refining, 198
    regulation of, 197–98
technology
    causa of objects of, xiii,
        41–43, 224,
        245
    conflict minerals in elec-
        tronic, 196, 199
    fear of, 247
    fixing problems of, 195
    hero status of, 241
    impact of modern, 87
    mining, 81–82
    replacing human systems
        with, 27–28
    resistance to new, 28,
        74–75
    safety of new, 185–86
Thomas, Katie, 177, 180
thrombus, 125
    See also blood clots
tin
    mining ore for, 39, 196
    regulation of, 197–98, 199
titanium
    in defibrillator can, 41, 45,
        47–48
    extraction of, 155
    products with, 148, 154, 168
    See also ilmenite
Tolstoy, Leo, ix
trauma, definition of, 194
treadmill test, 23, 27
Trump, Donald, 205, 209, 210

tungsten
    mining ore for, 39, 196
    regulation of, 197–98
Turner, Todd, 124

Uganda, mining and violence
    in, 196–98
ultrasound, 23, 115
United Nations General As-
    sembly, Kimberly Process
    of, 198
University Medical Center
    (Tucson, AZ), 165, 191,
    216
University of Arizona
    graduate program at,
        134–35, 135, 138
    teaching job at, 213, 214
uranium mining, 69, 167

vitamin K, Coumadin and, 122

wire extraction surgery
    approaches to, 234, 237, 246
    danger of skipping, 182–83,
        194–95, 237
    decisions about, 181–84,
        186, 208–10
    first, 187–94, 200, 238
    friendly advice on, 219–21
    insurance for, 205, 213,
        217–18, 222–23, 228,
        229, 235
    risks of, 182, 236, 239
    scheduling, 235
    second, 238–39

wire extraction surgery (*cont.*)
    surgeon's fee for, 212
    tests and consultation
        before, 230–34
wolframite, 196
World Bank, 77, 147

X-rays, chest, 121, 122, 234
    3-D, 236, 238

yoga, 2, 138, 185, 207, 219–20

Zika virus, 211
zircon, 146, 155

ABOUT THE AUTHOR

Katherine E. Standefer writes from a juniper-studded mesa outside Santa Fe, New Mexico, where she lives with her chickens. Her debut book, *Lightning Flowers,* was shortlisted for the J. Anthony Lukas Work-in-Progress Prize from the Columbia Graduate School of Journalism and the Nieman Foundation for Journalism at Harvard. Her writing appeared in *The Best American Essays 2016* and won the Iowa Review Award in nonfiction. She has been a Logan Nonfiction Fellow at the Carey Institute for Global Good and a Marion Weber Healing Arts Fellow at the Mesa Refuge. Standefer earned her MFA at the University of Arizona and teaches at Ashland University's low-residency MFA. As a trauma-writing specialist, she helps other writers birth difficult and important stories about the body.